Tanya Telfair Sharpe, PhD

Behind the Eight Ball
Sex for Crack Cocaine Exchange and Poor Black Women

Pre-publication
REVIEWS,
COMMENTARIES,
EVALUATIONS . . .

"*Behind the Eight Ball* addresses, in a direct and unflinching way, a problem the general media only covers at ratings time. In a professional and academic manner, it details suffering that few can imagine and lets those who experienced the hard times speak for themselves. This is a book that will educate anyone who reads it. It argues strongly for improved addiction intervention services for poor black women."

Michael Brimacombe, PhD
Associate Professor,
Department of Preventive Medicine and Community Health, New Jersey Medical School—UMDNJ

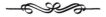

"This is an amazing publication that is a must-read for anyone who cares about the health of women, children, and our nation's families. It is obvious that the ten years of research that went into this document have been a labor of love for author Dr. Tanya Telfair Sharpe. She sheds light on an often misunderstood epidemic in our inner-city neighborhoods, addiction to crack cocaine, and the effects on black women and their families. Most compelling are the secret and tragic tales of the crack-addicted women who participated in her research. Their stories are gut-twisting, disturbing, and all too real. Dr. Sharpe was able to reach into the hearts and souls of women who have been ravaged by years of abuse, poverty, addiction, and neglect, and share their stories, helping the reader to see the multigenerational cycles of victimization and societal judgment. Thank you, Dr. Sharpe, for putting a face to the forgotten souls of addiction and reminding us to see these women as beautiful souls who deserve the nation's attention and support."

Kathleen Tavenner Mitchell, MHS, LCADC
Vice President and National Spokesperson, National Organization on Fetal Alcohol Syndrome

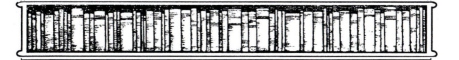

More pre-publication
REVIEWS, COMMENTARIES, EVALUATIONS . . .

"Tanya Sharpe's book is an incisive and insightful look at a group of women who are denigrated and misunderstood in our society. Through their stories, Sharpe takes us into the lives of poor black women who exchange sex for drugs. She examines the social context that provides them with few viable options and looks at the impact that crack cocaine has had on their lives, in particular how it has affected their sexual choices, sexual health, and child-bearing and rearing.

This book should be required reading for all persons who come into contact with female drug users, whether they are policymakers, law enforcement officials, health care professionals, social service workers, family and friends, or simply concerned citizens. It is incredibly easy for most of us to dismiss or disapprove of women who exchange sex for drugs. After reading this book, which puts faces and stories to this nameless epidemic and gives shape to poor black women's lack of choices, their struggles, and their heartaches, one is never able to think of them in the same way again."

Denise A. Donnelly, PhD
Associate Professor of Sociology,
Georgia State University, Atlanta

"This is certainly a thought-provoking and heartfelt book; it provides a unique combination of the human tragedy of addiction with the scientific strategies to address a genuine public health crisis. Dr. Sharpe has an ear for soul-stirring stories and a heart for social justice. The blend of well-grounded epidemiology and case studies of one of the most marginalized groups within our society makes this book a contribution to the fields of drug-addiction research and drug-treatment practice.

Students of public health, psychology, sociology, criminal justice, and anthropology will benefit from the careful recording of human tragedy reflected here. Despite the human degradation that is so well documented in this book, Dr. Sharpe moves beyond sensationalism and demonstrates how people transcend unimaginable circumstances."

Charles B. Collins, PhD
Science Application Section Chief,
Division of HIV/AIDS Prevention,
Centers for Disease Control and Prevention

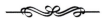

"*Behind the Eight Ball* is a fascinating new book that details the complicated life stories of women who use sex to support their addiction to crack cocaine. As a CDC researcher, Tanya Sharpe is especially well qualified to address the public health aspects of both unprotected sex and drug use. However, this book goes far beyond simply looking at the exchange of sex for crack as a public health crisis, and Dr. Sharpe assesses the practice in the context of racism, sexism, rape, the legacy of slavery, unequal power relationshps, and life in a dominant patriarchal culture. The personal stories these women shared with Dr. Sharpe are poignant as well as illuminating, and they provide intimate insight into a fascinating subculture that most of us will never directly experience. This is required reading for anyone genuinely interested in understanding this intractable social problem."

Danny Wedding, PhD, MPH
Professor of Psychiatry and Director,
Missouri Institute of Mental Health;
Editor, *PsycCRITIQUES: Contemporary Psychology—APA Review of Books*

More pre-publication
REVIEWS, COMMENTARIES, EVALUATIONS . . .

"In lucid prose, Dr. Sharpe describes the lives of poor black women who have fallen victim to another form of slavery: exchanging sex for crack cocaine. Professionals in health care, academics, and government will all benefit from this work. In providing a detailed analysis of the antecedents, a clear picture of the current crack culture, and the poor outcomes resulting from this vicious addiction, Dr. Sharpe has clearly advanced this field."

Mark B. Mengel, MD, MPH
Professor and Chair, Department
of Community and Family Medicine,
Saint Louis University School of Medicine

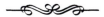

"Among those not involved in HIV-related health services and research, the fact that HIV is devastating black communities in this country seems to be tragically little recognized. Absent such recognition, cogent public health strategies cannot be formulated and effectively implemented. Reasons for the high rates of HIV disease in black communities are complex, having deep historical roots as well as a host of more recent socioeconomic influences. In her book, Dr. Tanya Sharpe investigates these issues both broadly and specifically: by a discussion of the evolution, or rather the devolution, of black communities in the United States from before the Civil War to the present, which then functions as background for the presentation of results of structured interviews with poor black women who exchange sex for cocaine. The picture that emerges is one of achingly desperate lives, of fierce power struggles between men and women in a context of economic and educational impoverishment amid drastic social upheaval. It is a harsh reality that is pictured here, but one from which we can no longer afford to avert our gaze—it needs urgently to be brought to light.

This excellent book is indispensable reading for anyone interested in gaining an in-depth knowledge of the complex issues affecting the spread of HIV in black, inner-city communities—a matter that should be regarded as of critical interest for all socially concerned Americans. The conjunction of Dr. Sharpe's extremely well-informed, scholarly approach with her evident compassion for the women she discusses and interviews has produced a highly compelling work, which will disturb—and rightly so—anyone with a functioning conscience. However, her book is more than a call to action; in its sensitive and detailed descriptions of women's lives racked by cocaine addiction, and in its specific recommendations for programmatic change, it makes a crucially important contribution to health services policy and HIV-prevention programs in inner-city neighborhoods."

Arthur Margolin, PhD
Research Scientist,
Department of Psychiatry,
Yale University School of Medicine

Behind the Eight Ball
Sex for Crack Cocaine Exchange and Poor Black Women

Haworth Psychosocial Issues of HIV/AIDS
R. Dennis Shelby, PhD
Editor

HIV and Social Work: A Practitioner's Guide edited by David M. Aronstein and Bruce J. Thompson

HIV/AIDS and the Drug Culture: Shattered Lives by Elizabeth Hagan and Joan Gormley

AIDS and Mental Health Practice: Clinical and Policy Issues edited by Michael Shernoff

AIDS and Development in Africa: A Social Science Perspective by Kempe Ronald Hope Sr.

Women's Experiences with HIV/AIDS: Mending Fractured Selves by Desirée Ciambrone

Hotel Ritz—Comparing Mexican and U.S. Street Prostitutes: Factors in HIV/AIDS Transmission by David J. Bellis

Practice Issues in HIV/AIDS Services: Empowerment-Based Models and Program Applications edited by Ronald J. Mancoske and James Donald Smith

Preventing AIDS: Community-Science Collaborations edited by Benjamin P. Bowser, Shiraz I. Mishra, Cathy J. Reback, and George F. Lemp

Couples of Mixed HIV Status: Clinical Issues and Interventions by Nancy L. Beckerman

Lesbian Women and Sexual Health: The Social Construction of Risk and Susceptibility by Kathleen A. Dolan

Behind the Eight Ball: Sex for Crack Cocaine Exchange and Poor Black Women by Tanya Telfair Sharpe

Behind the Eight Ball
Sex for Crack Cocaine Exchange and Poor Black Women

Tanya Telfair Sharpe, PhD

The Haworth Press®
New York • London • Oxford

For more information on this book or to order, visit
http://www.haworthpress.com/store/product.asp?sku=5175

or call 1-800-HAWORTH (800-429-6784) in the United States and Canada
or (607) 722-5857 outside the United States and Canada

or contact orders@HaworthPress.com

The Haworth Press, Inc., 10 Alice Street, Binghamton, NY 13904-1580.

PUBLISHER'S NOTE
Identities of individuals discussed in this book have been changed to protect confidentiality.

Cover design by Marylouise E. Doyle.
Cover photo of crack cocaine vial by Mark Kinsley.

Library of Congress Cataloging-in-Publication Data

Sharpe, Tanya Telfair.
Behind the eight ball : sex for crack cocaine exchange and poor black women / Tanya Telfair Sharpe.
    p. cm.
  Includes bibliographical references and index.
  ISBN-13: 978-0-7890-2456-5 (hc. : alk. paper)
  ISBN-10: 0-7890-2456-X (hc. : alk. paper)
  ISBN-13: 978-0-7890-2457-2 (pbk. : alk. paper)
  ISBN-10: 0-7890-2457-8 (pbk. : alk. paper)
    1. African American women—Drug use. 2. Poor women—Drug use—United States. 3. Narcotic addicts—United States—Sexual behavior. 4. Drugs and sex—United States. 5. Crack (Drug)—United States. 6. Children of prenatal substance abuse—United States. I. Title.
    [DNLM: 1. Cocaine-Related Disorders—ethnology—United States. 2. Crack Cocaine—United States. 3. African Americans—United States. 4. Poverty—United States. 5. Sexual Behavior—ethnology—United States. 6. Social Problems—United States. 7. Women—United States. WM 280 S532b 2005]

HV5824.W6S53 2005
616.86'47'008996073—dc22
                                                    2005003162

The Future
To my daughter: Lois J. Sharpe
To my niece and nephew: Whitney C. Watts and Elliot J. Watts

The Present
To my husband,
Claude W. Sharpe Jr.
and my sister, Tezlyn Telfair Watts

The Near Past
In loving memory of
Renaille Sharpe Daniels (1962-1999), my sister-in-law who died
of AIDS
Willie L. Telfair Jr., my father (1926-1988)
Lois Holley Telfair, my mother (1927-1968)
Louise Delaney Holley, my maternal grandmother (1900-1979)
Frank H. Holley Jr., my maternal grandfather (1902-1985)
Annie H. Telfair, my paternal grandmother
Willie L. Telfair Sr., my paternal grandfather

The Distant Past
Dedication to my ancestors:
Emma Delaney (1871-1922), my great-great-cousin,
Spelman College graduate, 1896, and a missionary to Africa, 1914

Dr. Joseph Holley (1874-1958), my great-great-uncle,
founder of Albany State University, Albany, Georgia

Bishop Henry Beard Delany, my great-great-cousin,
cofounder of St. Augustine College in Raleigh, North Carolina,
and father of Bessie and Sadie Delany

Thomas Sterling Delaney (1810-1890)
and his wife Sarah Elizabeth Delaney (1814-1891),
my maternal grandmother's great-grandparents

ABOUT THE AUTHOR

Tanya Telfair Sharpe, PhD, is Research Behavioral Scientist with the Centers for Disease Control and Prevention, Division of HIV/AIDS, Capacity Building Branch, Science Application Team. She serves as a science officer for diffusing evidence-based HIV-prevention interventions nationally. Dr. Sharpe coordinates science and technology transfer from universities and other research institutions to community-based organizations, and provides leadership on national HIV-prevention interventions' projects targeting at-risk youth and illicit-drug users. Dr. Sharpe's research interests include social inequality, maternal and child health, HIV/AIDS epidemiology, substance use during pregnancy, and urban studies.

CONTENTS

Foreword

I am proud to be associated with this book by former student and current colleague, Dr. Tanya Telfair Sharpe. It is a significant work that describes and analyzes a practice among some black women who are trapped in a debilitating cycle of inner-city poverty. The book also offers recommendations on how to positively address and change the socioeconomic conditions and public health policies that perpetuate the practice of poor black women selling sex for crack cocaine.

Some readers will be shocked to learn that women engage in unprotected sex, which subjects them to HIV and AIDS, in order to feed their addiction for crack cocaine. Others will be stunned to discover the extent to which the women who do so bring crack-addicted babies into the world—babies who must be cared for by relatives and friends because their mothers cannot care for them. Even those who are aware of the exchange of sex for crack cocaine will find in this book an unusually penetrating look into this sad and shameful reality in black urban life.

Drawing on a firm command of the relevant literature, and with insights from her use of both ethnographic and quantitative methods, at no time does Dr. Sharpe slip into blaming the victim of this practice of prostitution to support a crack cocaine addiction. Rather, she chronicles the social and economic changes in American inner-city neighborhoods that created optimum conditions for the distribution and consumption of crack cocaine. Dr. Sharpe carefully exposes how the triple marginalization of race, gender, and class combine to put poor black women disproportionately at risk for exchanging sex to feed a crack cocaine habit. The tragic consequences that individual black women experience are compounded in terms of negative effects on the children who are born to these crack-addicted women and the severe pressures put on the extended black family and child welfare agencies that must care for another generation who will be entangled in a web of poverty, drugs, and unfulfilled potential.

This book helps readers understand the similarities and the differences between traditional prostitution and exchanging sex for crack cocaine. In doing so, the author highlights just how male dominated crack culture is and the extent to which women are profoundly marginalized within it. Just as important, Dr. Sharpe lets speak "the invisible women" who are trapped in an unrelenting pattern of selling themselves to feed a drug habit, only to have to continue the exchange of sex for crack cocaine. Through the words of these women, readers hear how the circumstances of their lives—poverty, poor education, parental substance abuse, limited access to jobs, and unsatisfactory relationships with men—are an ideal setup for luring them into using crack cocaine. Once they are hooked on this drug the only means at their disposal for satisfying their habit is to sell themselves.

Absolutely nothing pretty exists in the picture of poor black women who are, as Dr. Sharpe puts it, behind the eight ball. It is a picture at which we must stare and endeavor to understand so that something can be done.

Dr. Johnnetta B. Cole, PhD
President of Bennett College for Women,
Greensboro, North Carolina;
President Emerita of Spelman College

Acknowledgments

This book is the culmination of more than ten years of work. Along the way so many people have supported and cheered me from the sidelines. I would like to recognize them for being there for me professionally and personally.

This book could not have been written without the women who generously opened their lives and shared their pain, suffering, disappointments, joys, and triumphs with me. I owe so much to them. I keep them in my heart and think of them often. Their faces are ever before me. These memories keep me focused on bringing their unique struggle to the forefront of the American public policy debates. The women I interviewed are intelligent, gentle, resourceful, and have unlimited human potential. They are beautiful, wonderful people who deserve a second chance. I thank them now, and I am committed to finding ways to help them and their children.

I could not have completed this project without the help of the late Faye Brown Sperling and of Pat Brown, Tony Childs, and Gwen Payne, who served as subject recruiters and advisers during the research process. Their knowledge, expertise, and willingness to help were greatly appreciated

I would like to sincerely thank the National Institutes of Health National Institute on Drug Abuse (NIDA) for providing me with a National Research Service Award (F31) to support the research. Dr. Leslie Cooper, my NIDA project official, was extremely supportive throughout the research process.

Dr. Donald Reitzes, chairman of the Georgia State University Department of Sociology, provided the infrastructural support for this project. The research and manuscript were strengthened by the help of a number of educators who reviewed early drafts. Dr. Denise Donnelly, who served as my adviser, is, without question, the best mentor a research fellow could ask for. She provided support and encouragement throughout the entire research process. Moreover, when I approached her with my idea to apply for a federal grant to support the project, she took a chance on me and agreed to serve as my sponsor.

She had faith in me and believed in me. I'll never forget her consideration and the time she shared with me. She also provided expert consultation on gender and sexuality, social inequality, and family studies. Dr. Phillip W. Davis and Dr. David Petersen provided consultation regarding qualitative methods and family violence, and substance abuse, respectively.

Many others at Georgia State University helped me in ways that they probably don't realize. I appreciate every courtesy extended to me by faculty members, departmental staff members, and administration staff members. Selma Poage, Quanda Miller, Robert Singleton, and Diedra Crockett were helpful and congenial also. These outstanding departmental employees made my research at GSU much more manageable. Ms. Esther Peters helped me greatly with the administration of my research grant. She is truly a shining star among GSU employees. Ms. Albertha Barrett, Darren Ingram, and Stephen Smith made the grant administration process much easier as well.

I am grateful to Dr. Johnnetta B. Cole, former President of Spelman College, Atlanta, Georgia, and current president of Bennett College, Greensboro, North Carolina, for serving as a consultant on this project. She provided expertise on black women and gender studies. Dr. Cole has been my role model for more than twenty-five years. She provided guidance and assistance personally and professionally in innumerable ways.

I have a number of friends at Spelman College who should be recognized for their kindness and encouragement. I have been able to count on Dr. Daryl White and Dr. Harry Lefever for more than fifteen years. They both provided encouragement, friendship, and support, which helped me persevere and complete the research. Mrs. Emma J. Redding at Spelman is another special friend. She was never too busy to listen when I needed a willing ear.

I would like to thank Dr. Claire Sterk, chairperson of the Department of Behavioral Science and Health Education, Rollins School of Public Health, Emory University, for providing me with the first opportunity to interview female crack users. When I served as research coordinator on her project titled Epidemiology of Drug Use Patterns Among Women with the Department of Anthropology at GSU, I interviewed female drug users for the first time. This experience changed my life. Before this I was not fully aware of the depth and severity of life challenges faced by female crack users. I would like to thank

Mark Kinsley of Yale University for the photograph used in the cover design.

Most important, my family stayed close to me throughout the years before and during the process of the research and drafting the manuscript. I would like to thank my dear sister and brother-in-law, Tezlyn and Ervin Watts, and their children, Whitney Watts and Elliot Watts, for their encouragement, support, and kindness. My dear stepmother, Julie Rivard Telfair, also deserves recognition. She is a cherished member of our family. I would like to recognize my brother, Frank Telfair, for always making me laugh.

I owe special gratitude to my beloved husband, Claude W. Sharpe Jr., and my beloved daughter, Lois J. Sharpe. They lived through this process with me step by step. My husband was very kind, understanding, and supportive. He also provided help with computer-related issues when I needed it. My daughter's sparkling presence gave me determination to finish the project.

Finally, and supremely important, I thank God. God gave me the strength to face all of the obstacles that confronted me, and provided insight and direction in finding paths to overcome them.

Introduction

The baby I am carrying now, I don't know who the father is.
There are a few [men] that I had sex with around the time I got
pregnant, that day. But which one it is, I don't know who.

A poor black female crack user

When asked to talk about this research I often explain that I didn't
choose this subject; it chose me! I interviewed poor black female
crack users for the first time in the summer of 1992, in the context of
the broader topic of the epidemiology of female drug use patterns.
Before that time I knew almost nothing about the plight of poor black
female crack users. However, after interviewing middle-class and
poor, black, white, and Hispanic female users of heroin, cocaine powder, and crack cocaine, it became immediately apparent the poor
black female crack users experienced the worst forms of social degradation and received the fewest opportunities for help. Even among
street substance users they were the most marginalized. Poor black
female crack users were disproportionately subjected to violence,
traumatized, raped, and they more often resorted to prostitution to
support their drug habits compared with other drug users. These are
the nameless, faceless women we hear about on the six o'clock news:
"body of unidentified black woman, age thirty-five to forty-five,
found in dumpster."

After hearing many of their soul-stirring stories, helping them became a calling in my life. These women have enormous human potential, intelligence, and resourcefulness rivaling many American
women of privilege. However, the social infrastructure and support
by which women of privilege obtain education, careers, spouses, and
opportunities for either self-sufficiency or family interdependence
are almost nonexistent for poor black women.

The findings of this study represent a small tip of a very large ice-
berg. Most poor black women first tried crack cocaine in social settings with friends, relatives, or the men in their lives (Henderson

et al., 1994; Williams, 1989). No one could have predicted the drastic changes that would occur in their communities and their lives because of one thing: crack cocaine. The women were encouraged to try it, initially, free of charge. Quickly the supply of free samples disappeared and the male drug dealers marketed it in small, affordable quantities (Williams, 1989). Many found that the crack-induced burst of omnipotence provided short-lived relief from deeply rooted feelings of inadequacy brought on by the effects of race, class, and gender exclusion (Bourgois, 1989; Devine and Wright, 1993). This feeling was desired again and again, and personal, professional, and public-assistance resources were exhausted. Having nothing left to trade, sell, or with which to bargain, the women's bodies became the commodity. Exchanging sex for crack, or exchanging sex for money to buy crack, became an integral part of the crack experience for many poor female users (Inciardi et al., 1993, Young et al., 2000, Sharpe, 2001). At first the drug was concentrated in the hands of high-level dealers who lived outside of their communities. However, the lure of fast cash attracted the masses of unemployed inner-city black youth to become highly organized drug entrepreneurs (Devine and Wright, 1993). This widened the pool of men willing to engage in sex for crack. This pool became wider as the price of prostitution dropped and the word spread to middle-class blacks, whites, and many others that sex could be obtained at budget prices from women who were addicted to crack (Young et al., 2000). Marginalized women, desperate for the drug, will engage in unprotected vaginal sex with many different men simply to gain access to quantities of the drug (Inciardi et al., 1993). A number of studies indicate that condom use is inconsistent among crack users (Kenen and Armstrong, 1992; Ratner, 1993). The dramatic rise in sexually transmitted diseases, including HIV infection and AIDS among urban poor blacks is evidentiary (Booth et al., 1993; Forney et al., 1992; Fullilove et al., 1992; Marx et al., 1990; Sterk, 1988).

Pregnancy is the other consequence of high volume, unprotected sex. It has been demonstrated that many women use crack during their peak years of reproductive proclivity (Substance Abuse and Mental Health Services Administration [SAMHSA], 2001). This book probes the complexities of exchanging sex for crack and its consequences among poor black female crack users. Exchanging sex for crack cocaine places women at risk for health complications and premature death due to HIV/AIDS and has changed pregnancy and childbearing patterns.

Human reproduction has historically existed within culturally prescribed behavior patterns and regulatory norms that serve to govern family formation and ensure the socialization of offspring. The sex-for-crack barter system that evolved after the introduction of the drug to inner-city neighborhoods has altered the previous processes and has resulted in serious consequences for the lives of poor black women and their children (Inciardi et al., 1993; Ratner, 1993; Mahan, 1996). These consequences include unplanned pregnancies, trauma from multiple miscarriages and abortions, and unwanted children who have slipped through traditional extended family safety nets. These outcomes initially impact the quality of life of the woman, and later impact society as well.

I view sex for crack and its consequences as empirical evidence of the multiple processes of long-term, consistent social exclusion and systemic racism that has worked to destroy poor black American women's sense of self-identity. A fundamental part of this identity assault comes from gender roles for black women developed in the context of slavery and segregation and based on erroneous concepts of black inferiority and a complicated dual sexual image, both asexual and hypersexual at the same time. Another part of the assault comes from the structure of American economic opportunity, which often unrepentantly relegates black women to the most basic roles. In addition, the wax and wane of the social policy toward blacks opened short-lived windows of opportunity for the privileged few, closing quickly and ever defaulting to the same rhetoric expounding "black undeservedness."

The devastating complications of crack cocaine addiction for poor black women are incompletely understood. The goal of this research is to extend beyond the sensationalism of sex-for-crack exchanges. Cultural understanding of this behavior as it impacts the sexual risk taking and the reproductive potential of individual women was sought. Specifically, this analysis sheds light on a neglected dimension of sex-for-crack exchanges and gives voice to the women who engage in this behavior. For many of these marginalized women, pregnancy and motherhood are among the few choices available that offer life satisfaction and self-validation (Kearney et al., 1994a).

Considering the controversial nature of the research, one could argue that any discussion of such explicit material is culturally insensitive since an unflattering picture of poor black female crack users may emerge. Similar arguments were leveled against the Moynihan Report, which foretold of the coming schism between poor and nonpoor blacks in 1965. Daniel Patrick Moynihan contended that initiatives to shore up poverty-stricken black families, who at that time had assumed the female-headed, single-parent family structure, should be a national priority. Moynihan's work became linked to Oscar Lewis's *La Vida* (1965) and the culture of poverty theory. Lewis describes the culture of poverty as a pathological subculture characterized by family disorganization, inadequate childrearing practices, substance abuse, the quest for immediate gratification of shortsighted goals, impulsive behavior, crime, and myriad other unfavorable stereotypes. Although Lewis's study concerned Latin American poverty, the theoretical scheme was widely applied to blacks and used interchangeably with Moynihan's. This unfortunate association obscured the true significance of Moynihan's findings and social and economic diversity extant within the black population. Nevertheless, the line between poor and black became blurred in the process and frequently "poor" became a euphemism for black.

Black and white scholars, rather than poor black families, rose in rebuttal to the unflattering depiction of "black" families. Chiefly using vignettes, these scholars emphasized the strengths and resilience of black families. Single-parent, female-headed households were considered creative, adaptive strategies that developed in opposition to the dominant hegemony (Billingsly, 1968; Hannerz, 1969; Moore, 1969; Liebow, 1967; Rainwater, 1970; Stack, 1974). The well-meaning attempts to shift the focus away from a negative depiction of any group of blacks was understandable at that point in time since resistance to social reform in favor of minorities was common. However, these events obscured the difficulties of the poorest subgroups of blacks for more than twenty years. Now, largely attributable to the geographic concentration of the poor in inner-city neighborhoods, the "tangle of pathology" described by Moynihan is unquestionable (Wilson, 1987; 1996). The aforementioned chronology of the controversy surrounding the Moynihan report clearly points to the need for nonpolitical objectivity in social research, even when sensitive issues are probed. This kind of candor in research is especially indicated now that the crack-cocaine proliferation has reached a zenith. Working from this vantage point, an analysis of sex for crack and its consequences is important for a number of reasons.

First, sexual risk taking in the context of the crack culture is well documented (Cross et al., 2001; Elwood et al., 1997; Hoffman et al., 2000; Inciardi and Surratt, 2001). I wanted to know what the women were thinking about when they engaged in vaginal sex without the protection of condoms and why they decided to have unprotected sex with strangers.

Second, given that many female crack users are of childbearing age and that many don't use birth control, I wanted to know if women were becoming pregnant in sex-for-crack exchanges. Furthermore, if they did become pregnant, I wanted to ascertain the outcomes of these pregnancies and the motivations behind decisions to abort the pregnancy or to keep the child. I also wanted to know the life circumstances of the children who were brought to term. Conceptions such as these may, in part, explain family disruption and the increase in the child abuse, abandonment, and neglect associated with women who use crack. Having children by prostitution clients may increase the likelihood that these children will have a geometric decrease in familial support at best, and at worst no family support. It has been demonstrated that the extended family system has been overwhelmed by a flood of children whose parents are addicted to crack (Minkler and Roe, 1993). It is not known, however, if sex-for-crack conceptions played a role in these displacements.

The behaviors of compulsive crack smokers have confounded conventional treatment providers, overwhelmed the social service industry, and shocked the nation with sensational stories of abuse and neglect, especially to children. The combination of irresponsible procreative activity and crack use plays a large part in the unhealthy socializing mechanisms that characterize many inner-city poor communities.

Third, the rapidity with which crack cocaine changed reproductive patterns underscores the women's vulnerability and the need for comprehensive and culturally competent strategies to address myriad social pathologies that plague them. This study provides evidence of the fragility of the social organization among the urban poor by demonstrating the powerful influence of a single agent as an instrument of social change, and it may call into question the current resurgence of biological-determinist explanations for social phenomena. Recently, scholars in the social sciences have resurrected arguments that were prevalent in the 1950s and 1960s concerning biological determinism and social decay (Murray, 1984; Rushton, 1996). They contend that genetic makeup predisposes racial groups for cultural, social, and behavioral patterns. These arguments are reminiscent of very early human classification schemes based on a vertical linear scale from higher to lower. Darker-skinned people were placed at the bottom of the hierarchy in terms of culture, social organization, and physical development; lighter-skinned people ranked at the top (Feagin and Feagin, 1993). J. Phillipe Rushton is a contemporary proponent of this perspective. His controversial 1996 journal article "Race, Genetics and Human Reproductive Strategies" outlines a linear classification scale that rates human reproductive patterns based on parental investment by race. Rather than using a vertical scale, his continuum is horizontal and places Asians at one end of the scale and people of African descent at the other. Caucasians fit squarely in the middle. He suggests that black people have more offspring and care for them less, and in contrast, that Asians have fewer offspring and invest more time and energy in their progeny. Whites are moderate parental investors. Furthermore, he argues that the propensity for nurturing children is genetically inherited (Rushton, 1996). These arguments minimally account for or neglect altogether cultural and social factors that mediate effective child nurturing. In addition, adopting a rigid, biologically based approach obscures the impact of extraneous social forces on the reproductive patterns of the inner-city poor. One such formidable force is the sex-for-crack phenomenon.

Fourth, the findings of this research add to the literature on sex for crack. Although issues such as the increases in sexually transmitted diseases linked to crack-related sex have been researched (Booth et al., 1993; Forney et al., 1992; Fullilove et al., 1992; Marx et al., 1990; Sterk, 1988), the relationship between sex-for-crack exchanges and pregnancy has not been addressed. The body of research and literature on reproduction and crack use has been limited to the following issues: crack use during pregnancy and intrauterine drug exposure (Bateman et al., 1993), the criminalization of pregnancy and fetal rights (Elshtain, 1990; Palthrow, 1990; Maher, 1990; Schedler, 1992) and teenage pregnancies (Marques and McKnight, 1991). Pregnancies conceived by sex-for-crack exchanges remain unexplored.

Fifth, this research adds as well to the literature on diversity extant in the black population.

A specific sociodemographic group known to have experienced race, class, and gender exclusion was chosen for this study. Alisse Waterston's (1993) research stresses the structural vulnerability of marginalized individuals and the relationship between the sociocultural system and drug addiction. Crack abuse can be seen as a symptom of a larger societal problem: the long-term neglect of the poorest subgroups of the black-American population. A number of crack-cocaine studies in the past have stressed the importance of racial and ethnic differences in the experiences of users (Bachman et al., 1991; Blanton et al., 1993; Gilmore, 1990). Most of the research samples drawn for these studies have come from isolated inner-city neighborhoods and are therefore overwhelmingly made up of poor black subjects among the "urban underclass" (Inciardi et al., 1993; Mahan, 1996; Wallace, 1991). (See also Wilson, 1987, or Devine and Wright, 1993, for detailed discussion of this demographic group.) Emphasis on race frequently overshadows social class.

Behavioral research on blacks in America has also been controversial. Models of ethnic and cultural diversity have rarely been applied to blacks, other than to distinguish them from other groups (Omi and Winant, 1994). The present study emphasizes the marginality and unique characteristics of poor black women as a gender group within a distinct subculture or social class. The participants in this research are not representative of the total black female population. Thus, the findings contribute to the knowledge of the heterogeneity of American blacks.

This book is the culmination of more than ten years of research on the socioeconomic changes in inner-city neighborhoods that created the optimum conditions for a crack stronghold, the crack-cocaine economy's impact on the lives of inner-city residents, and the social and familial consequences of crack addiction among poor black women. In addition to background research, I conducted short screening interviews with forty-six poor black women who exchanged sex for crack weekly or more frequently to support their drug habits, and I conducted in-depth, ethnographic interviews with a subset of nineteen women who became pregnant by exchanging sex for crack.

In rich, ethnographic quotes the women share the details of their lives before and after crack cocaine's introduction to their communities. They recount the circumstances of initiation into crack use and their first experience exchanging sex for crack. The women explain why they do not use condoms when exchanging sex for crack, share the motivations behind their decisions concerning sex-for-crack pregnancies, and describe the life circumstances of sex-for-crack–conceived children. The women's story, recounted in their own words, is an American tragedy that highlights the widening gap between social and economic classes.

Chapter 1

The Social and Economic Precursors of Crack Use in Inner Cities

Substance abuse is a frequently cited affliction of the urban poor (Anderson, 1978, 1990; Bourgois, 1989; Dembo, 1993; Devine and Wright, 1993; Inciardi et al., 1993; Ratner, 1993; Staples, 1991; Wallace, 1991; Williams, 1989; Wilson, 1987). Heroin and marijuana use have a long history of association with ghetto environments (Becker, 1953; Rosenbaum, 1981). In the past, users and distributors of drugs remained on the periphery of the social structure, however, the nationwide social and economic changes that occurred in the 1970s and 1980s changed the sociodemographic makeup of inner cities and set in motion rapid and progressive infrastructure decay (Divine and Wright, 1993; Wilson, 1987). These changes created the optimum structural conditions for a crack stronghold in inner-city neighborhoods (see Figure 1.1) (Dunlap and Johnson, 1992). Figure 1.1 visually illustrates, from bottom to top, the structural support for crack proliferation provided by the inner-city conditions described in this chapter.

First, the impact of the civil rights legislation passed in the 1960s opened channels of opportunity for educated and prepared black Americans. Acting upon these advances, middle- and working-class black people began an exodus from segregated inner-city neighborhoods in favor of better housing in suburbs. Stable families and those with moderate to strong mainstream connections were no longer stalwarts of the inner-city communities. The most economically and socially fragile ranks of black communities were left behind (Wilson, 1987, 1996).

Second, the economic transition to a highly technical service base, which shrank the pool of available low-skill, entry-level manufacturing jobs, and the relocation of factories to foreign countries and Ameri-

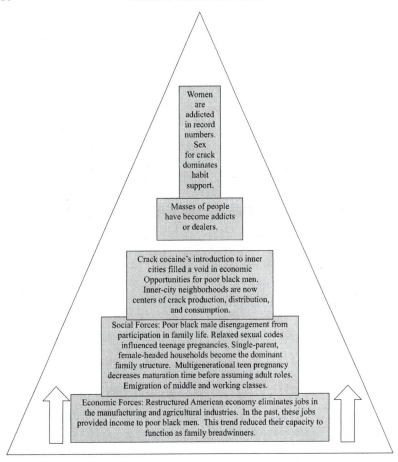

FIGURE 1.1. Social and economic precursors of crack cocaine use. Complex, interrelated social and econonmic forces created the optimum conditions for a crack cocaine stronghold.

can suburbs severely constrained and in some cases eliminated inner-city employment opportunities (Wilson, 1987; Devine and Wright, 1993). Concomitantly, the agricultural industries in the South became highly mechanized during the 1970s, decreasing the need for manual labor. Traditionally, displaced workers in rural agriculture found refuge in a plethora of blue-collar jobs available in urban manufacturing plants. In the 1970s, unemployed agricultural workers flooded inner cities at a time when plants were closing, relocating to suburbs, or moving to other countries. Thus, a large pool of superfluous, unskilled black male workers became concentrated in urban centers (Wilson, 1996). Unemployment for poor black males reached a critical mass in the early 1980s (Dunlap and Johnson, 1992). Absence of breadwinner jobs for men is traditionally linked to family instability and male retreat from responsibility among poor blacks (Anderson, 1990; Liebow, 1967; Moore, 1969; Stack, 1974; Wilson, 1987).

Third, the relaxed sexual codes of the 1960s and 1970s that emphasized sexual freedom for women and legitimized premarital sex had the unforeseen consequence of an explosion of teenage pregnancies among poor blacks (Wilson, 1987). Well-meaning social programs of President Lyndon Johnson's "Great Society" enabled unmarried pregnant teenage girls to drop out of high school, obtain subsistence income, and in some cases, low-cost housing away from their families. These trends established the female-headed, single-parent household as the predominant family composition pattern and exacerbated male disengagement from marriage and procreative responsibility (Stack, 1974; Staples, 1991a). Furthermore, multigenerational teen pregnancy shortened the years between generations, resulting in a change in age structure toward increased number of youth (Wilson, 1987). The ultimate result of the aforementioned social forces was the concentration and isolation of extremely young, socially and economically vulnerable individuals in circumscribed geographic areas. At this critical juncture, social policy toward blacks changed again in the early 1980s. Ignoring historical discrimination and the results of economic restructuring, a modern group of social Darwinists and neo-eugenics proponents such as Charles Murray (1984) and others suggested that the problems experienced by inner-city poor blacks were attributable to intellectual and cultural inferiority. Following the findings of these scholars, conservative politicians pushed to dismantle Great Society programs to aid and train the poor (Wilson, 1987). Into this volatile set of circumstances the crack phenomenon proliferated.

The final piece of this disturbing picture occurred in the early 1980s. Before then, cocaine was considered a recreational drug for the upper and middle classes. The cost of the drug was prohibitive for the poverty stricken (Williams, 1989; Dembo, 1993). That is, until the cocaine-producing countries (such as Chile, Bolivia, and Peru) experienced a cocaine glut that resulted in two consequences. First, stockpiled quantities of cocaine invited experimentation with ingestion methods. It was discovered that a smokeable cocaine precipitate could be produced by "cooking" cocaine powder together with baking soda and water. Smoking cocaine, rather than intranasal inhalation, was thought to prevent damage to the sinus passages and was found to produce a quicker and more intense high (Waldorf et al., 1991; Williams, 1989). The solid form of cocaine was called "crack" because of the crackling sound it made when smoked (Williams, 1989). Second, the diminished street value of powder cocaine influenced drug dealers to search for new markets for distribution. Free samples of crack were then distributed in inner-city poor neighborhoods and housing projects. With addiction assured, the dealers then marketed the drug in affordable five and ten dollar prepackaged quantities (Williams, 1989).

This clever marketing strategy dramatically changed the lives of the urban black poor economically, socially, and culturally. The inner-city poor were an attractive target for marketing the drug in this manner due to the predictable pattern of public-assistance delivery. A drug dealer need only appear in poor neighborhoods on or near the first day of each month when money from welfare checks became available. Furthermore, abandoned buildings in a deteriorating infrastructure were perfect locations to establish clandestine crack businesses. Unprecedented numbers of people became addicted, windows of opportunity opened for the masses of unemployed youth to become "dope boys" (community drug dealers), and inner-city neighborhoods became centers of drug sales and consumption, and in response the community's weak links to the mainstream of society have been nearly severed. As well, venerated social institutions such as the church and the extended family system that have supported impoverished blacks since slavery have been severely strained or dismantled completely (Staples, 1991).

CRACK USE AND WOMEN

Before the introduction of crack, illicit hard drug abuse was commonly associated with men (Anderson, 1978; Rosenbaum, 1981). In 1968, male substance abusers outnumbered women by a five-to-one margin (Rosenbaum, 1981). In the 1970s there was a slow but steady increase in female drug users of heroin and marijuana (Inciardi et al.,

1993). However, after the appearance of crack cocaine in inner cities, unprecedented numbers of women have become addicted (Inciardi et al., 1993; Ratner, 1993). The well-documented link between sexual activities and crack cocaine has complicated the lives of poor black women and their children (Anderson, 1990; Forney et al., 1992; Inciardi, 1989; Inciardi et al., 1993; Minkler and Roe, 1993; Ratner, 1993).

A disproportionate number of female crack users are poor and black (Bateman et al., 1993; Forney et al., 1992; Fullilove et al., 1992; Inciardi, 1989; Inciardi et al., 1993; Kearney et al., 1994a,b; Mahan, 1996; Maher, 1990; Minkler and Roe, 1993; Pursley-Crotteau and Stern, 1996; Ratner, 1993).

The 1997 Drug Abuse Warning Network (DAWN) estimates of drug-related visits to hospital emergency rooms suggests that crack smoking is a health problem for blacks in general and for black females in particular. In 1997, 18,114 women were admitted to emergency rooms for crack-related emergencies. Of these, 65 percent were black, 29 percent were white, and 6 percent were Hispanic. Black females outnumber white females more than 2-to-1 in crack-related emergency room visits (U.S. Department of Health and Human Services, 1997). The 2003 DAWN report indicates that cocaine related visits to emergency rooms increased by 36 percent (U.S. Department of Health and Human Services, 2003). The Drug and Alcohol Service Information System (DASIS) report, presenting 2002 data from the Treatment Episode Data Set (TEDS), reports that 73 percent of cocaine users admitted to drug treatment reported smoking cocaine, and among the smokers, 57 percent were black (U.S. Department of Health and Human Services, 2005). A different DASIS report dated July 13, 2001, indicated that a majority of adult women entering treatment for crack cocaine addiction in 1998, 61 percent, were black, compared with 33 percent white and 5 percent Hispanic women (U.S. Department of Health and Human Services, 2001).

This pattern is typical of Mitchell Ratner's *Crack Pipe As Pimp,* 1993. Based on aggregated data drawn from major cities in the nation, Ratner's sample of 340 subjects was 72 percent black and 69 percent female. Likewise, out of 14 female crack users in Fullilove and colleagues' 1992 study, 10 were black. Seventy-two percent of 68 women were black in Kearney, Murphy, and Rosenbaum's study on mothering and crack (Kearney et al., 1994b). In Pursley-Crotteau and

Stern's (1996) study of perinatal crack users, 81 percent of the 19 women were black. As well, 67 percent of the 27 adolescent females in James Inciardi's 1989 study population were black. Inciardi and colleagues' 1993 larger study on women and crack cocaine was predominantly black as well. In addition, all of the aforementioned samples were drawn from inner-city poor neighborhoods. This evidence supports a relationship between race, class, and gender marginalization and crack use. Cultural background and socioeconomic status are important variables that predict vulnerability to illicit drug use and the accompanying social devastation (Elwood et al., 1997).

Marsha Rosenbaum (1981) demonstrates this relationship in her groundbreaking study of female heroin addicts. She describes the phenomenon as a process of "narrowing options." As women become more involved in heroin use the chances for a stable home life, employment, and relationships with people who do not use drugs become increasingly scarce. Furthermore, Rosenbaum argues that minority women who use heroin have fewer life options to begin with (Rosenbaum, 1981). Similarly, her colleague Margaret Kearney argues that the narrowing of life options for female crack users is prevalent well before the onset of crack cocaine use (Kearney et al., 1994a). Following this line of reasoning, the impact of race, class, and gender marginalization among inner-city poor black women places them in a social position to be exploited by the male-dominated crack culture.

The set of dangerous behaviors associated with crack use has been especially damaging to poor black women due to chronic unemployment and the absence of meaningful social roles. Crack use is highly compulsive and leads users to spend large amounts of money over time by spending small amounts repeatedly until all resources are depleted. More affluent crack users may tap into larger pools of resources and have access to more material goods that can be liquidated if cash flow becomes a problem. Conversely, poor black women have limited income-generating power and fewer economic resources. Their sparse resources can be exhausted quickly by crack use. Furthermore, in the absence of careers outside the home, many are vulnerable to lapses in activity. The cycle of crack addiction fills the void in the lives of many disenfranchised women. Therefore, poor black women are disproportionately at risk for engaging in sex-for-crack exchanges to support their drug habits.

Exchanging sex for crack among poor black women is a complex issue for several reasons. First, women who exchange sex for crack are denigrated within the androcentric crack world. They are termed "hos," "skeezers," "strawberries," and a variety of other pejorative names (Fullilove et al., 1992; Elwood et al., 1997; Inciardi et al., 1993; Mahan, 1996; Ratner, 1993). Trading sex for crack has further emphasized their marginal position in society at large. More important, becoming a "crack ho" greatly diminishes gender-specific social power within their own communities by eroding the ability to function in culturally defined roles.

The prevalence of exchanging sex for crack as a means of habit support among economically deprived and socially isolated demographic groups that make up the urban poor is emphasized throughout published research reports (Forney et al., 1992; Fullilove et al., 1992; Inciardi et al., 1993; Ratner, 1993; Williams, 1989). These exchanges, characterized by higher levels of sexual activity and numerous partners, have been the subject of many studies (Fullilove et al., 1992; Inciardi, 1989; Inciardi et al., 1993; Mahan, 1996; Ratner, 1993; Williams, 1989). It is not unusual for crack-using females to engage in unprotected sex with anonymous partners in the genre of crack houses that have emerged (Ratner, 1993). These are houses, or more commonly, apartments in public housing where people can either purchase the drug, use the drug, engage in sex, or a combination of all three for various monetary charges. The compulsive nature of crack use leads to irresponsible risk-taking behavior during which condom use is inconsistent (Kenen and Armstrong, 1992; Ratner, 1993). The dramatic rises in sexually transmitted disease, including HIV infection, among the urban poor is a result of widespread crack addiction and the related increase in prostitution (Booth et al., 1993; Forney et al., 1992; Fullilove et al., 1992; Marx et al., 1990; Sterk, 1988).

Furthermore, the use of other contraceptives or prophylactic devices, for example birth control pills or diaphragms, is also inconsistent among crack users (Booth et al., 1993; Inciardi et al., 1993; Kenen and Armstrong, 1992; Ratner, 1993). Oral sex occurs most frequently among users on the street, however, vaginal intercourse is not uncommon (Inciardi et al., 1993; Ratner, 1993).

The repetitive cycle of "geeking and freaking," using crack (geeking), followed by performing sexual acts (freaking), followed by more crack use eventually consumes all or nearly all of the user's time. Crack-using women are constantly on the go for days at a time, either using crack, finding someone who will give them crack or the money to buy crack, or performing sexual acts until their bodies are exhausted (Miller, 1995; Muller and Boyle, 1996). This cycle makes it difficult for women to manage their bodies, their lives, and the lives of their children.

CRACK USE AND PREGNANCY

A majority of women who use crack do so during their child-bearing years (Kearney et al., 1994a,b; SAMHSA, 2001). This, in combination with high-volume, unprotected sexual acts, increases the likelihood of conception. Pregnant substance abusers in general are stigmatized (Murphy and Rosenbaum, 1997; Rosenbaum, 1981). Female crack users who become pregnant are perhaps the most stigmatized (Bourgois, 1989; Maher, 1990; Litt and McNeil, 1997). Pregnant crack users are depicted as monsters, shamelessly appearing in crack houses, purchasing crack, using the drug, and exchanging sex for crack, and often with babies or toddlers in tow (Bourgois, 1989; Hansen, 1998a; Litt and McNeil, 1997).

Pregnancy in and of itself is difficult for any drug-using woman and calls into play ambivalence concerning maintaining or abandoning the drug-user role in favor of motherhood (Kearney et al., 1994a,b). The mother is faced with a number of decisions. The two immediate options are abortion or carrying the child to term. The first option is relatively simple if emotional trauma is not considered. When pregnancy is terminated a woman may continue her drug-user lifestyle. The second option is more complex. If she chooses to carry the child to term, she must either confront her addiction or continue to use drugs to the baby's detriment. One source suggests that a common response to pregnancy is seeking drug treatment (Pursley-Crotteau and Stern, 1996). If the child is carried to term, a new set of decisions must be made, one of which is where to deliver the baby. Delivering a drug-exposed child in a public hospital or other health care facility may bring criminal charges (Maher, 1990; Palthrow, 1990, 1998; Siegel, 1997). Having a child elsewhere may be hazardous for the mother as well as the infant. After the child is born a mother must decide whether to keep the child, make an adoption plan, sell the baby on the black market, or risk losing the child through legal intervention.

The aforementioned factors are especially complex due to the social and cultural characteristics prevalent in inner-city poor black communities. Poor black women are the least likely to choose an abortion when faced with an unplanned pregnancy (Rainwater, 1960; Radecki and Beckman, 1992; Robbins, 1981).

This trend may be linked to religious concerns (Robbins, 1981) or the subtle influences from social undercurrents, such as fears of black genocide (Ward, 1986). Furthermore, having a child by an absent father may bear less stigma among the inner-city poor (Anderson, 1990). The demographic makeup of urban poor black families supports this conclusion. Limited social roles and career opportunities for inner-city women may influence decisions to keep children produced in sex-for-crack exchanges with the hope that deficits in their own social and emotional lives will be filled. Intergenerational teenage motherhood is probably another influence in the reproductive decision-making process. Burns and Burns' (1988) causal model of parenting dysfunction in chemically dependent women highlights the mothers' lack of parenting in their childhoods as a contributor to dysfunctional parenting in drug-addicted women. They argue that the lack of adequate nurturing in childhood carries a legacy that continues and grows as addicted women are faced with their responsibility of parenting. The change in age structure among the inner-city poor caused by the shortened years between generations (Wilson, 1987) has exacerbated the process of dysfunctional parenting by decreasing the amount of maturation time before the onset of childbearing. This phenomenon has reached extremes among poor crack-using females.

CRACK USE AND MOTHERHOOD

Children born to crack-addicted mothers have become a source of societal concern and research interest in recent years (Bateman et al., 1993; Elshtain, 1990; Kelley, 1992; King, 1991; Mahan, 1996; Maher, 1990; Marques and McKnight, 1991). Some of the key related issues that have emerged are (1) mothering while using crack (Kearney et al., 1994a,b; Pursley-Crotteau and Stern, 1996); (2) second-generation caregivers of children born to crack mothers (Minkler et al.,

1992; Minkler and Roe, 1993); and (3) intrauterine cocaine exposure (Bateman et al., 1993).

First, motherhood is extremely important to most poor women. However, balancing the roles of motherhood while addicted to crack is nearly impossible. The tension between the crack-user lifestyle and the responsibilities of mothering are often irreconcilable. The compulsive crack-use cycle and the self-centered experience of the crack high make self-sacrifice, nurturing, and focusing on the needs of children—which are characteristics of motherhood—difficult. Margaret Kearney and colleagues' (1994b) study of crack-using mothers found that the women in their sample placed high value on motherhood status and devised methods to separate their children from drug-use sessions, for example, by temporarily placing the children in someone else's care. Eventually, as the crack compulsion became stronger, these strategies were abandoned and the women lost custody of their children through family intervention or state-ordered foster care. Similarly, Pursley-Crotteau and Stern's 1996 study of perinatal crack users in drug-treatment programs for pregnant substance abusers suggests that their research subjects identified strongly with motherhood as well and used pregnancy as an opportunity to seek treatment. Delivery of a drug-free infant was the goal of the majority of women in their study. However, remaining drug free was dependent upon a combination of two positives: the personal desire to remain clean and a structured support system with sustained connections to mainstream life. The personal desire to stay clean was closely linked to identification with motherhood and acceptance of the pregnancy itself (Pursley-Crotteau and Stern, 1996). Women who were successful in the treatment programs understood the importance of creating distance between themselves and the drug-using environment. The absence of a drug-free support structure made it difficult for pregnant users to achieve the aforementioned goal.

These two studies shed light on the dilemma facing poor black female crack users. Most women want to be good mothers but find it difficult to achieve, even without crack. As mentioned before, they are often single parents, and have marginal education and few economic resources. Crack may provide momentary relief from these concerns. However, the saliency of being a mother for this group often reinforces the need for crack by increasing feelings of guilt.

The second research focal point related to crack use and motherhood is the increased pressure on the extended family system caused by crack-addicted mothers. Grandmothers, greatgrandmothers, aunts, and others have been overwhelmed with an influx of children who are under the age of five and were either abandoned by or forcibly removed from the custody of their drug-using relatives. In many cases these second-generation caregivers intervene on the behalf of the babies and young children for fear of their safety. Historically, the extended family provided safety nets for black children who lost parents under unfortunate circumstances. The breadth of the crack problem pushed this support mechanism to the limit by the sheer number of small children requiring care.

Minkler and Roe's 1993 study of black and predominantly poor second-generation caregivers points out the frustration and disappointment middle-aged and older women feel with second and sometimes third episodes of parenting. The few financial resources they possess, time, hopes for travel, and relationships with their husbands were lost in the process. The deep sense of duty they feel drives them to assume the responsibility, but many women are ambivalent about raising babies, toddlers, and preschoolers on fixed incomes. The findings of the study also support the notion of a change in age structure among the inner-city poor mentioned earlier and show how this change can decrease or lessen the support available for children. The ages of caregivers in the study ranged from forty-one to seventy-nine years.

Many of the women became grandmothers in their late thirties or early forties. Frequently, the older women in the sample were great-grandmothers or great-aunts. Younger grandmothers were occasionally unwilling to take on the responsibility of raising young children or may themselves have been involved with crack. In these cases, the responsibility shifted to the previous generation (Minkler and Roe, 1993). Under such conditions it is easy to understand why the child welfare system has assumed the responsibility for the many children who have slipped through the safety net of this overworked social structure (Lewis et al., 1997).

The third approach to the study of crack use and motherhood expressed in the literature is the focus on intrauterine cocaine exposure. Evidence suggests that significant numbers of poor black women who use crack do so during pregnancy (Bass and Jackson, 1997; Batemen et al., 1993). Early in the crack epidemic children born exposed to crack were described as developmentally challenged, hyperactive, aggressive, and devoid of human qualities (Kanteowitz, 1990; Toufexis, 1991). These reports, primarily by popular media, were based on anecdotal data and were unsubstantiated by empirical research.

The scientific research results on the effects of prenatal cocaine exposure are difficult to interpret because cocaine powder and crack are often used interchangeably (Bateman et al., 1993; Chasnoff et al., 1989; Woods, 1998). Moreover, distinctions made between modes of cocaine ingestion call into play demographic differences based on drug-use patterns and therefore American societal problems with race and class (Duster, 1997).

Cocaine powder users are primarily white and more affluent. Crack users are generally people of color and poor. These factors often discourage open discussion of uniqueness associated with crack use. Concomitantly, the resurgent school of biological determinism stresses alleged genetic deficits among poor blacks to explain the negative effects of crack cocaine. Literature based on state-of-the-art research suggests that cocaine powder and crack cocaine are very different in their pharmacological and biological effects. A number of scientists suggests that the by-product, produced when cocaine is smoked (or burned) rather than snorted, MEG (methylecgonidine), may be linked to irreversible damage in fetuses as well as irreversible damage to women who smoke crack (Scheidweiler et al., 1999).

Ronald Wood and colleagues (1996a,b) demonstrated MEG caused irreversible heart and lung damage to laboratory animals in vitro and in vivo (Hassan and Wood, 1995; Wood et al., 1996a,b). They observed acute heart-lung toxicity and structural damage in squirrel monkeys and guinea pigs. In addition, when pregnant ewes were injected with the substance, acute effects to the fetuses were observed (Wood, 1999). Furthermore, this group of scientists discovered that MEG was also capable of producing a Michael Addition reaction. This means that MEG is capable of forming covalent bonds with suitable moieties found in the body (Scheidweiler et al., 1999; Wood, 1999). If MEG is capable of bonding with body compounds then it could possibly bond with brain chemicals, for example, dopamine.

Crack cocaine is known to interfere with normal dopamine metabolic processes in the brain (Kreek, 1998). The aforementioned research raises many questions concerning the pharmacological and biological effects of crack that could possibly change behaviors.

Equally important is the research conducted by behavioral scientists suggesting that the poverty environment and neglect due to the mother's drug use are as likely as prenatal crack cocaine exposure to produce the psychosocial behaviors in children described previously (Hansen, 1998a). Some researchers suggest that growing up in the disorganized and dangerous home of a crack-addicted mother is more detrimental to the development of children than in vivo crack exposure (Hansen, 1998a,b,c,d,e). Again, the link between poor social and economic conditions and crack use is emphasized. These conditions have been exacerbated by widespread and pervasive crack use.

Crack use during pregnancy is associated with preterm births. Black women in general are more at risk for delivery of preterm and low birth weight babies (Green, 1994). Poverty and malnutrition are known to contribute to preterm births (Green, 1994). However, this trend is made much worse by crack use during pregnancy (Bateman et al., 1993). The combination of crack exposure and prematurity leaves children with neurological, respiratory, and other long-term health problems—if they survive the first six months of life in a less-than-conducive environment for child rearing (Bateman et al., 1993).

THE ATLANTA CRACK SCENE

Social and economic structural changes that transformed cities in the North and West occurred later and proceeded more slowly in the urban South. Cities in the eastern Sunbelt were able to hold on to their manufacturing bases somewhat longer than those elsewhere. Atlanta literally became a boomtown in the late 1970s in terms of economic growth (Orfield and Ashkinaze, 1991). The city of Atlanta is a model of the paradoxes in race relations and class struggles in American society. Atlanta emerged in the media as a mecca for the black middle class and a city "too busy to hate" with relatively good race relations (Jaret, 1986, p. 65; Orfield and Ashkinaze, 1991, p. 5).

However, the economic expansion in manufacturing and retail industries was disproportionately located in the nearly all-white north suburbs, for example Cobb and Gwinnett Counties. Whether the people followed the jobs or the jobs followed the people is not clear, but between 1970 and 1980 the white population in the city of Atlanta shrank by 44 percent (Orfield and Ashkinaze, 1991).

By the mid-1980s Atlanta's economy shifted to the now familiar bipolar postindustrial service pattern. A host of technical, government, and prestigious information-age jobs were created. Jobs in the center city were either highly technical, requiring high skills, or were the very low-pay, low-skill, dead-end variety. Fast food work is one example. Significant numbers of whites continued to move to the suburbs and commute to the city to occupy the newly created high-paying jobs. However, certain groups of highly educated, professional whites preferred to remain citybound in upscale areas such as Midtown, Inman Park, Virginia Highlands, Candler Park, and East Lake (Orfield and Ashkinaze, 1991).

Many middle-class blacks found jobs in the private sectors of this booming new economy but many more gained employment in the federal, state, and local governments. Middle-class blacks began a steady exodus to the nearby suburbs in south Fulton and south Dekalb Counties. The transition of these areas to a nearly all-black population was swift as white flight took its toll. Concomitantly, public policy toward housing for the poor placed multiple-unit government housing projects in or near these black neighborhoods. These complexes were used to house the thousands of poor blacks displaced by the urban renewal initiatives that gave Atlanta its first stadium and interstate highways (Orfield and Ashkinaze, 1991). Although civil rights legislation, in theory, opened the door for fair housing, continued segregation was supported by this complicated interplay between individual and government decisions. These demographic changes concentrated a disproportionate number of poor people in segregated pockets of the center city and nearby suburbs. Concentrating large numbers of extremely poor people in these neighborhoods contributed to their decay. Another contributing factor to the decay of some of Atlanta's core neighborhoods was the suburbanization of entry-level jobs.

Increasingly, the better-paying, low-skill jobs with future potential were concentrated in the northern suburbs. By 1985, manufacturing jobs in the suburbs outnumbered those in the city by a 2.5-to-1 margin (Orfield and Ashkinaze, 1991). Thus, as Stephanie Coontz (1992), has characterized other cities, Atlanta has a "spatial mismatch" between jobs and jobholders. Inner-city poor residents with few marketable skills could benefit from the manufacturing jobs still available in the suburbs but did not have the transportation to get to them. The counties with the most available low-skill jobs, Gwinnett and Cobb, have been most resistant to any expansion of public transportation, in any form, to their boundaries (Orfield and Ashkinaze, 1991).

Scholars disagree on whether Atlanta had actually become a center for black middle-class prosperity. In fact, some studies indicate that blacks at all education levels have not benefitted equally with their white counterparts from Atlanta's economic growth. Charles Jaret's (1986) study suggests that despite the plethora of jobs created by the postindustrial economic reorganization, middle-class blacks have not reached parity with whites in terms of income or occupational standing (Jaret, 1986). Jaret cites black overrepresentation in low-paying market subsectors, for example, personal services such as hotels, restaurants, hair care facilities, and the like, and white overrepresentation in the extremely high-paying financial-services subsector as contributors to the income differentials. Similarly, Sawicki and Moody (1997) point to increased numbers of immigrants to Atlanta who absorb the better-paying low-skill jobs, leaving blacks, especially young, unskilled black males, with fewer opportunities. Nevertheless, the public relations campaigns emphasizing Atlanta as a good place for black achievement influenced migration from two socioeconomic backgrounds. The promise of high standards of living and good jobs attracted emigration to Atlanta by well-educated blacks from the north and west after cities declined in those areas. These individuals were likely to occupy middle-class jobs and settle in suburban areas (Orfield and Ashkinaze, 1991). The final groups of displaced agricultural workers were also attracted to Atlanta. These unskilled individuals likely settled into inner-city poverty.

Atlanta has thus become a city with a split personality. On one hand it is a center for information-age technology with a thriving private- and public-sector postindustrial economy. On the other hand, it has extremely segregated, very poor sections of town with collapsing infrastructures, low tax bases, high unemployment (especially for unskilled, young black males), and poor-performing schools. Similar to many other poverty-stricken areas in the country where black males have difficulty obtaining earning power, single-parent, female-headed, welfare-dependent households predominate. In this highly segmented architecture, the crack cocaine epidemic has mushroomed.

One of the first articles on crack appeared in the *Atlanta Journal-Constitution* on June 27, 1986. Interviews with law enforcement officers indicated that the first documented cases involving crack occured that year. Few police officers had ever heard of crack at that time. This article also suggested that no large-scale crack-distribution networks existed, rather there were "thousands of small dealers out there pushing drugs" (Thomas, 1986, p. C-1). This is consistent with many sources (e.g., Williams, 1989; Jacobs, 1999) concerning the marketing of crack that emphasize the ease with which independent entrepreneurship is entered into at varying distribution levels. The underground economy of crack marketing fills the vacuum created by the spatial mismatch of jobs described earlier.

By 1988 crack had encroached into nearly all of the poor sections of town. Drug sales and use were especially concentrated in government housing projects. Crack-related crimes proliferated. The violence associated with crack use and sales, such as open drug dealing and drive-by shootings, reached a zenith at the Bankhead Courts housing project. Utilities companies, public transportation, and even the U.S. Postal Service temporarily stopped servicing the complex for fear of the open gunfire often experienced there (Gelb, 1990). Also in 1988, the staff at Grady Memorial Hospital suspected that "a new drug was affecting Atlanta's newborns" (Hansen, 1998a, p. A-1; Schwartzkopff, 1990, p. A-6). Grady serves the inner-city poor and indigent. These staff members saw a dramatic increase in babies requiring neonatal intensive care. Eventually, tests would reveal that crack cocaine was the culprit. To everyone's horror, social service workers at the hospital discovered that women and girls were using crack cocaine throughout their gestation (Schwartzkopff, 1990). In February 1989, 30 percent of babies in the neonatal intensive care facility at Grady tested positive for cocaine (Schwartzkopff, 1990). Unprepared for the deluge of babies born exposed to crack and without a systematic strategy in place to cope with these medically fragile children, many were sent home with their drug-addicted mothers (Hansen, 1998a). Forty percent of babies born to crack addicts at Grady were released from the hospital to their mothers (Hansen, 1998c).

By 1990 the Atlanta area's schools were preparing to receive a cohort of these children in public school kindergartens. Teachers and administrators anticipated the worst and predicted that many children would be mentally, physically, and/or emotionally handicapped due to fetal crack ingestion (Schwartzkopff, 1990). When more information became available, growing up in the home of a crack-addicted mother was cited as more damaging for children than the actual drug exposure. Many children are frequently left at home alone with no adult supervision and are provided inadequate diets. They are at risk for early death from a number of causes, the leading of which is abuse or neglect (Hansen, 1998a).

A little more than a decade after the epidemic began, crack use had tapered off in many major cities in the United States. However, in Atlanta, the phenomenon has continued and evidence suggests that crack addiction is spreading among poor black women of childbearing age (Hansen, 1998a) (see Figure 1.2). In 1997, 81 percent of women ages 26 to 30 arrested in Atlanta tested positive for cocaine. Furthermore, Atlanta statistics from the National Institute of Justice indicate that prostitutes as well as women age 31 and older were also more likely to test positive for cocaine when arrested. Eighty-five percent of female arrestees testing positive for cocaine were charged with prostitution (Hansen, 1998a).

The women in the studies were predominantly black and poor. (Hansen, 1998a). These figures suggest that Atlanta is experiencing tremendous growth in young-adult black women using crack and a strong relationship between addiction and exchanging sex for crack. The same social devastation characteristics of other major cities associated with crack addiction, such as increased crime, vagrancy, homelessness, and prostitution, are present in Atlanta as well. Grandmothers and other older women have taken on the parenting of small children abandoned or neglected by crack-using parents (Hansen, 1998e).

Social services have been overwhelmed by numerous children with no place to call home, and the soaring costs of caring for these very sick, premature babies born to crack mothers are absorbed by the hospital or taxpayers. With the help of teenage pregnancy, a full two generations have now grown up in the crack culture since the mid-1980s (Hansen, 1998a,b,c,d,e).

The crack culture and its related violence, devastation, and changes in family organization in inner cities is not only connected to the shifting tide of public policy; it is also rooted to patterns of ambiguous gender roles for blacks that developed during the social and economic upheavals occurring in the United States since slavery. Chapter 2 offers a historical analysis of gender roles among blacks that contributed to and supported the development of roles for black women in the crack world.

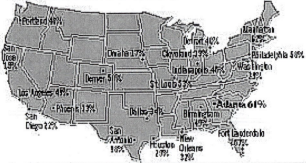

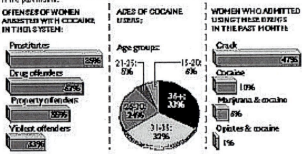

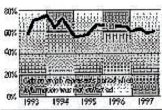

FIGURE 1.2. Female crack users in the Atlanta area. *Source: Atlanta Journal-Constitution,* September 27, 1998, "Growing Up with Crack" series by Jane Hansen (Hansen, 1998a).

Chapter 2

Bearing the Legacy of Social Change: A Theory of Gender Roles Among the Inner-City Poor

GENDER ROLE ORIGINS

For black Americans, family formation and gender roles were developed with severe social and economic constraints imposed upon them by institutional racism. These constraints did not remain constant over time. Rather, the ebb and flow of social policy toward blacks by the dominant culture required flexibility in self-definition and gender role differentiation. Blacks have faced a series of four abrupt social changes that necessitated rapid restructuring of gender-based identities and roles: (1) enslavement, (2) manumission and segregation, (3) civil rights legislation and desegregation, and (4) late-twentieth-century reverses in civil rights policy.

These transitional periods were not weathered equally by all. Certain groups of blacks have consistently benefited less from social policy designed to eliminate racial discrimination than others. Following the literature through the aforementioned periods, a clear trail of evidence exists that lends support to the theory of poor black dislocation and economic displacement expounded by William Julius Wilson in his book *The Truly Disadvantaged* (Wilson, 1987). At the same time, social and economic structures can be found that exert pressure on males and females to conform to gender roles inconsistent with mainstream models. This chapter offers a gender role theory that connects the structural dynamics of American racial policy to gender role development among the extremely poor. The earliest black experiences and circumstances, the division of slave labor, the personalities of slave owners and slaves, and perhaps random chance charted many blacks on courses that would make it difficult for them to gain and

maintain mainstream economic and social viability. With each subsequent transitional period, many blacks were estranged from access to
any mechanism (for example, education, job skills, firsthand knowledge of mainstream white culture) that would serve as a bridge to
economic self-sufficiency.

This chapter is presented with a caveat. The research on the black-
American family and gender roles is problematic. A dichotomy of research foci exists in the literature. The plethora of studies has focused
either on the black elite or the black poor. Not much is known about
those who exist in the middle of this continuum. Concomitantly, the
research on the poor frequently overshadows research on other socioeconomic groups among blacks, and the connection between black
and poor has been tenacious over time. Indeed, the term *poor* is sometimes used euphemistically for *black*. Unraveling the complexities of
black life is made more complex because of this tendency. The abundance of literature on the poor has dominated influence on public policy geared toward blacks with little regard to the experiences of middle and working classes. The theory herein works through the historic
experiences of blacks in general and narrows to explain the prevalence of specific gender role patterns among only the most disadvantaged socioeconomic groups. In the historic account, a pattern of isolation and marginalization of these disadvantaged groups, much more
so than other groups of blacks, will be shown.

SLAVERY AND GENDER ROLES

The first social change, the institution of slavery, imposed artificial
gender identities on blacks based on white men's perceptions of black
manhood and black womanhood. Furthermore, the conception of
blackness as a marker of ethnicity and cultural heritage was a Euro-
pean construction as well. When black Africans were first brought to
American shores, the definitions of manhood and womanhood in
their respective cultures did not apply in the new world. The ancient
traditions and principles of social organization were not only unrec-
ognized, but these individuals from diverse cultural backgrounds
were expected to live together in forced communities and share a
common identity based on their assumed inferiority (Noel, 1968). In-
digenous ascribed and achieved statuses and roles were eliminated
during the middle passage. The overarching condition of skin color

reduced all black Africans to distinctions between only male and female. At the beginning of their history in the American colonies, roles for black men and women were based upon the biological differences between the sexes, and highly sexualized notions of gender roles developed.

Angela Davis (1995), bell hooks (1981), and Paula Giddings (1984) assert that the construction of gender roles for black women began with the sexual exploitation of slaves. Using text from slave narratives, the aforementioned black feminist writers reconstruct the female slave experience and provide evidence that sexuality and procreative ability frequently defined social rankings among female slaves and made them targets for rape by white masters. In addition, nonconsensual pairings between slaves directed at producing more chattel were ordered by masters as well. For many female slaves, control over their own bodies was left behind on the continent of Africa.

Black women during this time were characterized as sexual temptresses or whores (hooks, 1981). Furthermore, according to hooks (1981), the sexualized identity rendered black women powerless against white men's advances and was a symbol of black men's powerlessness to protect them (hooks, 1981). Gender roles for men were sexualized as well. Black male slaves could achieve recognition and affirmation in two areas: exertion of physical strength and the siring of offspring (Frazier, 1939; Staples, 1970). These extreme stereotypes facilitated the characterization of black women as sex objects and black men as rapists. In general, most blacks were affected by these stereotypes, however, the degree to which they impacted their lives varied.

During enslavement, black people were not only caught between two sets of conflicting cultural norms, neither of which were self-determined, but were also subjected to dramatic differences in norms within their own ranks. Mainstream, white gender role norms that emphasized the male as provider and authoritarian figure and the female as homemaker and paragon of virtue existed in opposition to the gender role stereotypes for slaves that emphasized the male as the physically strong-but-obedient stud and the female as the always sexually receptive breeder. Making matters even more complex, the black experience before the Civil War was remarkably varied dependent upon slave or free status, geographical location, and the division of slave labor. Social stratification among blacks shaped experiences during the plantation economy and was instrumental in ushering them into antebellum lives. It is difficult to apply a strict class-based system to blacks during this period in the classic Weberian sense. Life chances and market opportunities for all blacks were limited by race at that time. Stratification is suggested in terms of quality of life, relative privilege, and access to the ruling-class cultural nuances.

The division of labor on plantations gave rise to a privileged class of blacks who were house servants and the field hands who were not so fortunate. House servants had a closer association with the white ruling class, often living in the same house. These slaves often had access to education and were allowed to acquire skills and trades. The house servants were more likely to adopt the speech patterns of the masters, giving them an advantage in terms of communication skills. The field hands lived further removed from the ruling class and therefore were more isolated from mainstream white society. These individuals were much more likely to develop the speech patterns known as the "Negro dialect" as their only language, which severely limited their mainstream communication skills. They had little access to educational opportunities and were seldom taught trades and skills that would have placed them in a better position after emancipation (Frazier, 1939, 1957).

One of the enigmatic features of the antebellum South was the presence of free blacks in urban areas. In cities all over the South lived 250,000 free blacks, many of whom were skilled artisans and craftsmen. These free persons, engaged in such businesses as bookbinding, cabinetmaking, brick masonry, architecture, and other such skilled occupations, made up a sort of "upper class" (Frazier, 1957; Wilson, 1978). After emancipation, free blacks were naturally in a better position than most slaves to weather the period of social and economic transition. They had more experience in functioning within the structure of the Southern society and had many contacts in the business community (Frazier, 1957).

As previously mentioned, the house servants were better educated than their field-hand counterparts, had marketable skills, were able to communicate and associate with whites, and understood the structure of white society. These slaves often had paternalistic relationships with their owners and received a certain degree of protection because of these associations (Feagin and Feagin, 1993).

The most disadvantaged groups of blacks were the field hands. Without education or skills they were in the worst possible position to enjoy freedom. Free blacks and house servants had better means of channeling themselves into the new economic system, having had greater exposure to the dominant culture (Blackwell, 1975). The unskilled, untrained, and isolated field hands had little recourse other than to become manual laborers and sharecroppers after emancipation.

The division of labor on plantations and resulting differentiation in types of skills further influenced the status ranking among slaves in determining the market value of the chattel. Slaves proficient in specific occupations, for example, blacksmithing or sewing, commanded a higher price on the auction block than did the unskilled. Moreover, those in the slave-trade business advertised the specific skills, using them as marketing tools (Katz, 1968).

Additional differences existed in the experiences of slaves residing in rural and those living in urban areas. Slaves in urban areas frequently had more freedom of movement, were more skilled, and were generally less closely supervised by whites. These slaves added to the ambiguity of the slavery system as they interacted with non-slave-holding whites, whose roles were also unclear under this economic system (Wilson, 1978). Urban slaves were often similar to indentured servants. They were frequently allowed to work for several people simultaneously and to earn wages. Portions of these wages were surrendered to owners, but these slaves were able to save some of the fruits of their labor for themselves (Sowell, 1994; Wilson, 1978). Urban slaves were in an enviable position after manumission, similar to that of free blacks. They commonly had established careers and a working knowledge of the mainstream white social and cultural nuances.

There were, in sum, four broad types of different experiences for blacks. In descending order of privilege, they were free blacks, urban slaves, plantation-house servants and skilled workers, and field hands. These structural parameters and status rankings mediated absorption of extremes in gender role characteristics.

A dichotomy of gender role stereotypes blossomed based upon ascription to mainstream cultural values. In 1939, E. Franklin Frazier's controversial book *The Negro Family in the United States* was published. Frazier, a student of Robert Park and Ernest Burgess at the University of Chicago, concluded that the lived experience of slavery shaped family formation and gender-specific roles for blacks before manumission. Using a wide range of qualitative data from plantation records, slave narratives, autobiographies of slaves and free blacks, accounts of visitors to the United States during the era, documents such as correspondence between overseers and slave owners, and published historical accounts, he formulated an assimilation theory.

According to Frazier (1939), blacks who had closer association with the dominant culture and those who had more favorable relationships with their masters assumed a patriarchal family pattern and mainstream gender roles based on variants of the two-parent nuclear family. Urban slaves, who had much more freedom of mobility than those on plantations, and house servants developed social organization and family structure similar to the white slaveholding ruling class (Frazier, 1957). Under these conditions, marriage among slaves was the norm, although the female role in the marriage was complicated by her dual role as slave. Slave women bore the additional burden of balancing care for her family with her responsibilities in the master's household or at her other place of employment. Role conflict in this context reached extremes if the female slave held the position of "mammy" in the master's household. Frazier explained that the mammy cared for the pregnant mistress of the plantation during the gestation period and served as a wet nurse for the white child beginning at birth. Furthermore, mammies were surrogate mothers for the master's children until they reached adulthood (Frazier, 1939). Caring for the children of the master's family constrained the amount of time that the mammy could devote to the nurturing of her own children (Frazier, 1939). Behavioral norms for slaves precluded the visible manifestation of this conflict in the work environment, but Frazier suggested that the slave family suffered the full impact of sharing wife and mother with the master's family (Frazier, 1939).

Despite the relatively favorable conditions of urban or house-slave status, the black male role as head of the family was truncated by the white master's ultimate authority over the entire family (Frazier, 1939). The married male slave could not assume the patriarchal role as sole family breadwinner in either the urban or plantation contexts. As mentioned previously, the married female urban slave was expected to work outside her home and the married female plantation house servant played a critical role in the maintenance of the master's household as cook, laundress, mammy, and so on. Moreover, the married male slave could not prevent the sale of members of his family if the master decided upon this course of action. Therefore, the male role within the slave two-parent family was eclipsed by the white male role as master and owner of the slave family.

Plantation field hands experienced slavery differently from urban or house slaves. They were isolated from the house slaves and whites in sexually segregated living quarters and subjected to more inhumane treatment, often through the efforts of a non-slaveholding overseer. As a group, the field hands have been described as more dependent and dominated by the harsh conditions of their existence. Equal work yields were expected for both males and females. Pregnant women and new mothers were not exempt from these expectations. Furthermore, distinctions were made between young women of childbearing age who were designated as "breeders." These women were frequently forced to mate with males not of their choosing in order to increase the slave population. Some males were relegated to "stud" or "stallion" status toward this end as well. This reproductive strategy was not conducive to emotional bonding between male and female partners and encouraged disengagement of males from family responsibilities.

The economic and social constraints and structured organization on large plantations left only two areas for the black male field hand to achieve self-esteem: sexual prowess and physical strength (Frazier, 1939; Staples, 1970). The field hand slave experience is characterized by sexual exploitation of slaves and partner selection by the ruling class. The male role of sire emerged as a primary source of life satisfaction for male slaves, as production of offspring was favorably acknowledged by plantation masters (Frazier, 1939; Staples, 1970).

The link between biological fatherhood and self-esteem was problematic for stable family formation among the field workers. The short-term goal of impregnation eclipsed the long-term responsibility of child rearing. Disruption attributed to slave sales was another hindrance to family stability. Since the sale of slaves was at the discretion of the master, the black male had little influence over keeping his family intact. This further diminished his status within the family. The other area in which black males could receive recognition was by exhibiting great physical strength as a prolific field worker. According to scholars, the female-headed household and male gender role marginalization developed within this subculture (Blackwell, 1975; Frazier, 1939; Staples, 1970).

Therefore some of the gender roles for field workers were developed by the masters for reproduction purposes only, similar to procedures for mating livestock. Frazier contends that the link between mother and child was the sole basis for family stability and that this social organization was the precursor to the self-defined black matriarchy. Moreover, he traces the postemancipation development of single-parent households, characterized by high rates of illegitimacy, to the former field hands on large plantations who later became sharecroppers (Frazier, 1939).

Thus, a bipolar notion of black gender roles was developed dependent upon proximity to the white culture. If blacks lived in close proximity to whites, they were mammies and uncles. The feminine role of mammy is characterized as asexual, self-sacrificial, long suffering, and at the same time domineering (Hill Collins, 1991). The masculine role of uncle was considered asexual, docile, bumbling, long suffering, and passive. On the other hand, if blacks lived further removed from the ruling class, they were characterized as highly sexual, dangerous, and morally deficit. These unflattering stereotypes persisted in the twentieth century (Hill Collins, 1991). The strength of Frazier's (1939) argument rests on highlighting the social isolation of the plantation field hands and distinguishing them as the most disadvantaged group within a disadvantaged race.

Among the free black population, some wives were required to work outside the home as well, and the patriarchal pattern of female concentration in unskilled, low-wage work was common (Frazier, 1939). However, wealthy, free black families who owned slaves patterned themselves closely after the Southern aristocracy. Females took charge of household duties and males functioned as family breadwinners (Frazier, 1939). The families of free blacks, urban slaves, and house servants assumed some form of mainstream family structure and gender role differentiation.

To summarize Frazier's treatise, the social order created by slavery in the South produced unique, gender-based relationships for black men and women. Status rankings among blacks in the plantation economy can be conceptually linked to family structure. Among the aristocratic, slaveholding, free black families, the patriarchal, male-breadwinner–dominated family structure was the norm. At the other end of the spectrum, field hand family structure was described as matriarchal. Moderately affluent free blacks, urban slaves, and house servants assumed variants of an egalitarian two-breadwinner family structure.

Frazier's (1939) continuum was put under fire by Herbert Guttmann (1976). Guttmann's study of the black family in slavery and beyond also challenged Frazier's (1939) most fundamental findings. Guttmann argued that no significant difference in family structure existed between house servants and field hands. Furthermore, he contended that the prevalence of the female-headed household among field hand slaves was exaggerated (Guttmann, 1976). His data indicated that, in general, slave women were expected to have children by one man, that the names of fathers were given to sons, and that families were more stable than commonly thought. Guttmann also suggested that serious methodological flaws in Frazier's (1939) analysis of the historical data cast doubt on his conclusions (Guttmann, 1976). These comments were issued after Frazier's death in 1962, so a rebuttal was impossible. Guttmann's work was heralded by black scholars as debunking the myths concerning the prevalence of female-headed households among slaves (Dill, 1990).

Guttmann's polemic with Frazier highlights the problematic nature of research on black Americans. In searching for the definitive interpretation of the black experience, the extensive variety of experiences was obscured. One of the serious flaws in Guttmann's analysis is one common to much of the research on blacks in America. Guttmann's data were drawn from a single segment of the slave population: those who lived on large plantations.

As indicated earlier, the experience of slaves on large plantations was not necessarily representative of the entire black population during the era. Furthermore, all large plantations were not organized and administered in the same way. To be sure, on the large plantations studied by Guttmann (1976), marriage and male-headed households probably were in the majority, irrespective of the division of labor. Frazier (1939), on the other hand incorporated data triangulation into his study and collected data from a variety of sources, which should reflect a wider range of experiences. Both scholars agree that plantation field hands were to some extent more segregated from whites and other blacks. They both find a consensus by stressing the importance of the extended-family system as a support mechanism and by emphasizing the importance of motherhood and female roles for family stability.

Taking both Frazier and Guttmann's perspectives together, the conditions of slavery produced four dimensions of gender relationships that influenced social interaction and family structure during segregation and later. First, in nearly all social rankings among slaves and free blacks, females did not develop dependency on black males for economic survival. After manumission, black females traditionally had higher levels of participation in the workforce than their white counterparts (Dill, 1990; Frazier, 1939; Guttmann, 1976; Lewis, 1977). Second, the male role as breadwinner was overshadowed by white male dominance of the economic system. Moreover, the mainstream standards for masculine roles were nearly impossible for most black males to live up to. The juxtaposition of the economic realities of black slave families against the upper- and middle-class white mainstream family economic conditions created a double standard of values that could not be reconciled (Frazier, 1939; Guttmann, 1976). Third, the conflict between the gender norms of the larger culture and the gender norms of blacks created tension between black males and females, with female family roles often overshadowing male family roles. Fourth, in some contexts, the sexual exploitation of field hands as studs and breeders may be directly related to more relaxed attitudes toward sexual activity, procreation, and parenting in this subgroup. Artificially constructed gender roles based on maximizing work efficiency and biological functions reached extremes among the field hands on large plantations.

The reduction of males and females to sires and breeders, respectively, disengaged men from long-term family involvement and shifted the responsibility of child support to the mother, under the institutional support of the plantation system. Furthermore, an extremely sexualized gender role identity emerged for both men and women in this context.

SEGREGATION AND GENDER ROLES: SIGNIFICANCE OF THE SHARECROPPING SYSTEM

The second social change, manumission, required blacks to make another adjustment to abrupt social restructuring. The formerly free blacks, urban slaves, house servants, and field hands were regrouped to form black communities, structured by the emergent Jim Crow segregation laws that racially polarized the South and established the official policy of racial exclusion (Franklin, 1969). Segregation in housing created black neighborhoods made up of individuals with different experiences and perspectives (Wilson, 1978). Male and female slaves instantly lost their institutional roles and faced the monumental task of finding mechanisms of support. Confounding matters, blacks witnessed the livelihood-enhancement benefits that were denied to them extended instead to the newly arriving white immigrants. An example of this was the Homestead Act. Some weathered the transition better than others. Marketable skills, access to education, and knowledge of the mainstream social organization and economic values were beneficial in this effort. As indicated before, these skills were clustered in specific slave occupations and statuses.

The privileged found their way into jobs in the emergent black community infrastructures and institutions. Females found access to work much easier than men. Domestic jobs in white homes became a primary source of income for many black women. In their experiences with the larger culture, the sexualized stereotypes followed them. A number of accounts suggest that black women working in white homes as housekeepers or cooks were subjected to sexual advances by their male employers (hooks, 1981). Males also had difficulty overcoming their sexualized images. The image of the brutal black rapist in the mind of whites made it difficult for black men to secure employment. Black male unemployment fueled the tension between men and women. By far, the newly freed slaves with the fewest options were the former field hands. Many of them were forced into sharecropping.

In this newly constructed society the two-parent nuclear family became the most prevalent structure of black families (Franklin, 1969; Guttmann, 1976; Sudarkasa, 1996). However, an estimated 20 to 25 percent of blacks families were single-parent, female-headed households between 1868 and 1960 (Sudarkasa, 1996).

Family structure and gender roles during segregation have been the subject of numerous studies on the black family (Bernard, 1966; Frazier, 1939; Herskovits, 1941; Johnson, 1934; Lewis, 1955; Moynihan, 1965; Rainwater, 1960). The prevalence of female-headed households among some segments of the black population, specifically the poor, became the principal concern of black-family scholars. Black families composed of married couples were not adequately researched during the segregation period. Two perspectives emerged to explain the persistence of the female-headed household family structure in the poverty-stricken portion of the population: (1) the influence of slavery and (2) the legacy of African cultures. As mentioned earlier, Frazier (1939) held that the matriarchal family was a product of the slave system and emphasized the position of blacks within the slave hierarchy as a determinant of this family structure. Moreover, the field hands on large plantations were linked to matriarchal family organization more than other groups of blacks, and they had fewer economic options in the immediate years following manumission. The sharecropping system that absorbed the majority of the unskilled field hands was an extension of de facto slavery. Under this oppressive system, significant segments of the most disadvantaged former slaves continued to be isolated from the mainstream black and white societies, similar to the conditions during plantation slavery. Male desertion of families among sharecroppers was common, reinforcing the prevalence of female-headed households (Frazier, 1939). Frazier argues as well that casual sexual relationships and widespread illegitimacy are legacies of slavery that persisted in the subculture that evolved among rural black sharecroppers. These explanations are echoed by Johnson (1934), who found similar patterns of family structure among black sharecroppers.

The postemancipation sharecropping system prolonged the experience of slavery and isolation for many field hands and continued the development of a subculture based on fluid conjugal pairings and capricious male involvement in family life. The connection between the sharecropping system and family structure is important for understanding the challenges facing the inner-city poor. Disadvantaged groups of black slaves were channeled into a de facto slavery after manumission and became entrenched in the sharecropping system. Agricultural work extended the lived experience of slavery for many blacks and prevented access to education and other upward-mobility mechanisms. The dynamics of isolated sharecropper existence produced gender roles for women that were, in some cases, consistent with the previously mentioned stereotypes (Johnson, 1934). Casual sexual relationships and widespread illegitimacy were common among black sharecroppers (Frazier, 1939; Johnson, 1934). Such behavior and sexual codes reinforced the negative images of the black female harbored by the dominant culture. Black female sharecroppers were frequently victims of rape and abuse by black and white men (Mann, 1989).

Though Frazier's (1939) slavery analysis dominated the field until the 1960s, another challenge to his thesis was suggested by Melville Herskovits. Herskovits (1941) contended that female-headed households among poor blacks were linked to the survival of African matrilineal-descent patterns. Furthermore, Herskovits argues that black male and female egalitarian breadwinner roles and female independence is a survival of African traditions also (Herskovits, 1941).

The question of the survival of African traditions among American blacks continues to interest more recent researchers. Niara Sudarkasa (1996) compared the historical traditions and gender role construction among West-African societies and African-American societies. She argues that the extended family system among blacks is a strong tradition in West Africa that has survived in America. Furthermore, Sudarkasa suggests that the importance of children, regardless of the marital status of their parents, is perhaps another cultural characteristic that has African roots (Sudarkasa, 1993). Conversely, Sudarkasa stresses that poverty-stricken, female-headed households, living autonomously without extended family support, is unknown in West Africa in the past and the present. Furthermore, she contends that most of the West-African tribes who were the source of slaves in America were patrilineally organized. Sudarkasa's (1993) findings cast doubt on Herskovits' (1941) analysis. Others have suggested that the survival of West African cultures was reduced by the sheer variety of cultures from which the slave population was drawn, and that it was discouraged by slave owners for fear of resistance movements (Noel, 1968). Regardless of whether the female, single-parent household began in America or Africa, the pattern persisted among the poorest segments of the black population and followed them as they emigrated from the South.

Lured by opportunities in the developing manufacturing industries in the North and West, a slow but a steady stream of black farmworkers migrated to cities beginning in 1900 (Wilson, 1978). Blacks who migrated to cities in the first waves fared the best. The expanding industries were able to absorb the majority of these unskilled workers. However, by the 1940s and 1950s emerging economic trends would prove disastrous for those remaining agricultural workers in rural areas.

Technological advances in farming replaced the need for human sharecroppers. As the displaced workers migrated to cities they found that the once-plentiful manufacturing jobs were also on the decline (Wilson, 1978). Urban areas in response became inundated with unskilled or semiskilled former sharecroppers at the same time that the economy was shifting to a polarized, highly technical, white-collar and extremely low wage service base. The development of an urban underclass can thus be linked to the extension of de facto slavery for blacks in the South who became entrapped in the sharecropping system and suffered from displacement as agriculture became mechanized, and who arrived too late to cities to benefit from the jobs created by the manufacturing industries in the first half of the twentieth century. These latecomers brought the legacy of the field-hand experience with them, a legacy of sexual proclivity and physical strength as markers of masculinity and motherhood and promiscuity as markers of femininity. The urban ghetto subculture and gender role structure of the 1940s and 1950s was rooted in the aforementioned phenomena (Blackwell, 1975; Frazier, 1957; Staples, 1970; Wilson, 1978, 1987).

The urban ghetto subculture has been the subject of numerous studies (Anderson, 1978; Bernard, 1966; Hannerz, 1969; Liebow, 1967; Lewis, 1955; Moore, 1969; Rainwater, 1970; Stack, 1974). Based on the culture-of-poverty thesis, the subculture is described as a pathological social organization pattern characterized by family disorganization, substance abuse, inadequate child-rearing practices, the quest for immediate gratification of shortsighted goals, impulsive behavior, crime, and myriad other unfavorable stereotypes. Oscar Lewis's (1965) original culture-of-poverty study concerned Latin Americans. However, the thesis is commonly applied to urban poor blacks.

During the last thirty years of segregation, black neighborhoods in urban areas were socially complex. In today's terms, they would be designated as mixed-use neighborhoods. Blacks of varied cultural perspectives and socioeconomic levels lived in close proximity to one another. Although the larger white society considered black neighborhoods to be monolithic, based on race alone, there were sharp social and cultural differences. The studies on urban black life conducted in the 1950s and early 1960s reflected the social stratification.

Two studies conducted during the era of segregation attempted to explain the social and cultural diversity that was extant in black communities. Both Hylan Lewis's *Black Ways of Kent* (1955) and Jessie Bernard's *Marriage and Family Among Negroes* (1966) highlight the complexities and paradoxes of black life before desegregation. Lewis describes the distinct cleavage in the community that he studied that resulted in two styles of life: the respectable and the unrespectable. The respectable lifestyle is characterized by work ethic, marriage and a two-parent family pattern, obedience to the law, and family stability. Conversely, the unrespectable lifestyle is associated with sexual promiscuity and illegitimacy, family disorganization, and trouble with the criminal justice system (Lewis, 1955). Similarly, Bernard found that black family structure in the township that she studied was based on orientation toward traditional or nontraditional value system. Furthermore, both researchers conclude that orientation toward mainstream norms cut across economic and education levels, though higher concentrations of the nontraditional strand clustered within the lower socioeconomic statuses.

Lewis's (1955) unrespectable and Bernard's (1966) nontraditional elements became the primary focus of social research to the exclusion of the respectable and traditional components of black communities. Eventually, labels such as the "culture of poverty" and "ghetto" were attached to those who did not fit mainstream models of behavior. It is important to note that widespread illegitimacy, family disorganization, and crime were held constant by segregation and forced housing policies. So-called "ghetto" blacks lived close to black teachers, lawyers, doctors, businesspersons, and ministers. Moreover, institutions such as churches and schools were often community refuges to which children from disadvantaged backgrounds could come in contact with positive role models. A genre of social and public service clubs in black communities, for example, lodges such as the Masons, Elks, and others; burial leagues; race-betterment clubs; and self-help societies all functioned to stabilize communities, help the needy, and attend to day-to-day community concerns (Frazier, 1957, 1969; Lewis, 1955).

Churches often functioned in this capacity as well. Black churches were much more than religious organizations. They served as educators and established missions to aid the elderly, the orphaned, and those in slums and in jails (Frazier, 1957, 1969). Church and denomination membership often served as identity markers for many blacks during segregation. Churches offered principal gender-based roles for men and women. In some denominations (Baptist, for example) men and women could achieve status by serving as deacons, deaconesses, elders, and mothers of the church. The mother of the church was of particular importance. This status was conferred upon an older woman of excellent character with many years membership in a church. She served as a mother figure for the entire congregation, and was referred to as Mother by all. Her choice of pew was generally unofficially reserved as her place and respected by the church members (Frazier, 1939).

A neglected dimension of black life during the period of segregation is the extraordinary nature of elementary and secondary black schools. These schools may have been economically disadvantaged, but the strength and high quality of the educators and administrators who worked at these institutions is greatly overlooked. Teaching and school administration were considered some of the most prestigious occupations a black person could hold at the time, and these positions attracted the top scholars. Moreover, it was not unusual to find people with advanced college degrees working at elementary, junior high, and high schools. This phenomenon offered the most disadvantaged black child opportunities for mentorship that are today unequaled in kindergarten through twelfth grade education. People informally educated in life experiences served as role models as well. These *Old Heads,* or oldest head in the neighborhood, were older men of character who shared the benefit of their wisdom and folkways with the younger generation. Old Heads were disciplinarians for their children and others in the neighborhood. In this way they served as guardians of the peace and order in the neighborhood (Frazier, 1939). Some older women functioned in the role of community mother or grandmother. Patricia Hill Collins stresses that these *Other Mothers* took responsibility for children other than their own and used kinship terms when referring to neighborhood children (Hill Collins, 1991).

The aforementioned role models, organizations, and institutions contributed to a cohesive though stratified black community that exerted pressure on the community to keep the unrespectable or nontraditional adherents on the periphery of society. Furthermore, these stabilizing forces acted to keep the roles for men and women balanced.

THE DESEGREGATION ERA:
PROLIFERATION OF A GHETTO SUBCULTURE
AND INCREASED GENDER ROLE TENSION

The third social change occurred during the desegregation era. Studies on urban black life at this time reveal more pervasive ghetto-related behaviors (Anderson, 1978; Hannerz, 1969; Moore, 1969; Rainwater, 1970; Stack, 1974). It is not surprising that these studies were conducted in the mid to late sixties and in the seventies when the unforeseen consequences of desegregation were first felt. The niches created for black businesses shrunk, and black entrepreneurs widened their marketing strategies to include other neighborhoods.

Stable, middle-class families began to leave inner-city neighborhoods, and with them went the tax base for the support of black schools. The highly educated black teachers could now apply for jobs at formerly all-white colleges or seek jobs in corporations. As opportunities opened for the privileged, options narrowed for the disadvantaged (Wilson, 1987). Poor black men were affected by these changes more rapidly than were black women. When they lost their jobs they lost the ability to function as breadwinners. To make matters more complex, the relaxed sexual codes of the larger society conveyed by the media legitimized early sexual experimentation among poor black teenagers, resulting in dramatic increases in out of wedlock births (Staples, 1991a,b).

Female-headed households, which were now more numerous and more geographically concentrated, again became the focus of research on the black family. The changing nature of male and female relationships in the poverty environment became a focal point as well. More specifically, the empowerment of women through access to money from work or access to resources from public-income transfers added to the tension between men and women. Tension between black males and females escalated due to increased gender role ambiguity for men and the black female independence that developed during this period. Although poor black women often made less money than their employed male counterparts, women could often count on jobs more consistently than males. Unemployment for poor black males grew worse after desegregation (Lewis, 1977). Moreover, public-income transfer programs such as Aid to Families with Dependent Children (AFDC) were accessible to only women under most circumstances (Hannerz, 1969; Staples, 1991a,b). Social-intervention strategies facilitated female independence by enforcing no-marriage rules for benefit eligibility (Hannerz, 1969; Staples, 1986). The shift in the balance of power between men and women set new standards for male-female relationships.

In a patriarchal society the male is designated as the family bread-winner, decision maker, and leader. Poor black males have had difficulty assuming this position within the family structure. However, the white male standards for masculinity, which emphasize power through economic success, are pervasive in American culture and constantly remind poor black males (and females) of the inadequacy of their performance as family providers. Acceptance of the mainstream ideals in combination with the structural constraints on economic opportunities and the slavery-derived sexual and physical definitions of masculinity have all contributed to an ambiguous position for poor black males in the family.

William Moore (1969) describes this phenomenon as masculinity without status. This ambiguity resulted in conflict with poor black women in two areas: (1) male retreat from marriage and family responsibilities and (2) sexual exploitation. These two issues are closely related, however, the latter may be viewed as a consequence of the former.

The poor black male retreat from marriage is a common theme in literature on the subject of poor black families (Anderson, 1978, 1990; Hannerz, 1969; Liebow, 1967; Moynihan, 1965; Moore, 1969; Rainwater, 1970; Staples, 1991b; Sudarkasa, 1996; Wilson, 1987). The lack of breadwinner jobs is generally cited as a primary influence on declining marriage rates (Massey and Denton, 1999; Wilson, 1987). According to a number of sources, the peer group became more important than marriage for ghetto men (Anderson, 1978; Liebow, 1967; Hannerz, 1969). Males in this setting frequently shunned conventional family life and opted for the classic street-corner lifestyle described earlier. The lifestyle is described as the everyday interaction among unemployed black men on city street corners.

This lifestyle has been the subject of numerous studies (Anderson, 1978; Bowman, 1993; Hannerz, 1969; Liebow, 1967) and is a persistent pattern among poor black men. These men find solace in banding together to discuss their sexual exploits, and view the traditional roles of husband, father, and breadwinner as emasculating and in a derisive manner (Anderson, 1990). Furthermore, they drift in and out of sexual relationships with women as a means of accessing economic resources and obtaining shelter (Anderson, 1990; Wilson, 1978). Without monetary means, men frequently employ various presentation-of-self strategies, such as style of dress, grooming, looks, dancing skill, and rap (conversation) to attract female interest (Anderson, 1990).

Though men attached themselves to women as an economic survival tactic, money from women's employment and the welfare checks were legitimately owned by women. Women, then, were established as the primary controllers of the economic resources flowing into these communities due to their access to public assistance, and this access was often mediated through her ability to produce offspring. Motherhood provided power in terms of procuring income, peer-group acceptance, and established the woman as the family breadwinner. The men, however, cultivated and used their powers of manipulation to benefit from female sources of income. Therefore many male-female relationships in this context were defined as exploitative (Anderson, 1990). Furthermore, family composition was subject to change periodically as new relationships were established and old ones terminated. These factors made family stability difficult. Although marriage began to decline among the poor, biological motherhood and fatherhood continued.

Poor black women in the first twenty years after civil rights legislation harbored mainstream ideals about marriage and family life, but their lives did not reflect their expectations (Staples, 1994). Marriage may not have been a realistic possibility, but becoming a mother was something most could count on. Poor black women took motherhood seriously. This may have been the single most important event (or events) in their lives (Staples, 1994). Motherhood was a source of pride and accomplishment when life offered little else. Becoming a mother was a rite of passage into adulthood, signaling to the community that the girl is now a woman (Anderson, 1990).

Anderson (1990) describes the *baby club* as a peer group of inner-city poor girls who have settled for the consolation prize of having a baby in lieu of marriage, for which the prospects are dismal. Becoming pregnant and assuming a welfare recipient's roles are methods of distancing oneself from inadequate families of origin and establishing adult status. For these girls, motherhood is supported at two levels. The peer group affirms the role and the society sanctions the role with financial support from public assistance. Thus, motherhood offers a source of status and life satisfaction by providing income and approval from peers. Furthermore, motherhood is a means of self-definition. Having children, caring for them, and rearing them are deeply connected to poor black women's self-worth and worth among her peers. Consider the following quote from a woman in Ulf Hannerz's (1969) study, *Soulside: Inquiries into Ghetto Culture and Community.* The following quote sums up the ghetto mother's plight, hard pressed by poverty but taking pride in her motherly accomplishments.

> A mother just got to fight for her children. It's hard if you ain't got no money and your man steps out on you, it's real hard. But you got to struggle, no matter what, 'cause they need you. So you got to be sure they got something to eat and something to put on and don't get into no trouble, and you make them understand that no matter what they can always come to mama. And you know, that's hard on you when you ain't got nobody to go to, when there ain't nobody to help you out, so you got to earn some money and raise a family too, . . . When you've worked all day long and you've taken care of the kids and they're in bed and you can just sit down or maybe go over to some neighbor for a game of whist or something, then you really feel good, 'cause you know what ever you've done, you've done your best. (p. 95)

Hannerz (1969) emphasizes that the poor black mothers he studied characterized themselves as near martyrs since they often bore family responsibilities alone.

Similarly, Carol Stack's (1974) study, *All Our Kin: Strategies for Survival in a Black Community,* demonstrated the importance of mothering for urban poor black women. The women in her study, whether married or unmarried, regarded child begetting and childbearing as a source of achievement and pride. For Stack's female research subjects, having children and raising them was preferred to any relationships with men (Stack, 1974).

Fatherhood without the benefit of marriage was a source of conflict in the inner-city poor environment. Nearly all of the ethnographic monographs on the inner-city poor conducted before the 1980s contain components that detail the unique dimensions of fatherhood (Anderson, 1978, 1990; Hannerz, 1969; Liebow, 1967; Moore, 1969;

Rainwater, 1970; Stack, 1974). The decline in marriage complicated the relationships between men and women and between fathers and children. Though a man's status in his family of origin (his mother's family) is clearly defined, his status in a family of procreation (his children's family) is determined by the state of his relationship with the children's mother. The indefinite article "a" is used in conjunction with family of procreation because a man may have more than one of these families. He may have children by several different women and not share residence with any of them. Moreover, he may reside with a woman whose children are not his and function as their surrogate father. The roles associated with boyfriend replaced those of the husband, and since this relationship may be temporary, fatherhood is often ambiguous for many inner-city poor men (Liebow, 1967; Moore, 1969; Rainwater, 1970).

David Schultz (1978) developed a typology of boyfriends among poor blacks based on the longevity of their relationships and extent of their economic support of female partners. His model consists of four ideal types.

First, the *quasi-father* is described as a boyfriend who has a long-term (five or more years) relationship with a woman but no biological children with her. He serves as surrogate father to her children by other men, and though his relationship with the woman is fairly stable, he has the freedom to come and go as he pleases. He provides significant contributions to the family income. Second, the *supportive biological father* is a boyfriend who has sustained stable relationships with his offspring produced by one or more women. Though his economic support of and relationship with his children is long term, conflict may occur if he shows preference or favor to the children of one household over others. Third, the *supportive companion* is described as a man in search of sexual gratification and free from responsibility. His economic support for a woman is largely token. If the woman has children by others, he is not likely to establish a relationship with them. Furthermore, this type of boyfriend will probably flee if he impregnates the woman. The fourth type of boyfriend is the *pimp,* who is analogous to a gigolo. His sole interest in a women is to harvest her income from welfare or wages (Schultz, 1978).

Similarly, Lee Rainwater distinguished between two types of boyfriends in the lower-class black social organization: the *good boyfriend* or the *pimp* (Rainwater, 1970). Rainwater suggests that even the good boyfriend's contribution to the family is marginal and benefits the boyfriend more than the family. His small contribution to the household pays for the right to be a pseudo family member (Rainwater, 1970). Conversely, the pimp times his visits when the public-assistance checks arrive. The pimp trades his companionship for food or money (Rainwater, 1970). These typologies demonstrate that even under the best circumstances, the roles of fatherhood are assumed at the discretion of the man, mediated by his current conjugal relationship, and not driven by family responsibility or the best interest of children.

Fluid conjugal relationships frequently produce children by different fathers in one household. This phenomenon is problematic for the woman, the man, and especially for the children. Fathers of one or some of a woman's children may be better providers and more involved in family activities than others. Conflict takes the form of jealously and rivalry among siblings, struggles between the man and woman if his contributions are shared with children by other men, and antagonism between the woman and noncontributing fathers (Moore, 1969).

Family compositions of this nature are stressful for children. Children by different fathers in one household may suffer from varying degrees of economic deprivation (Moore, 1969). Furthermore, maternal and paternal grandparent involvement may vary dramatically, depending on financial constraints, family structure, and the relative amity between the children's parents. Relationships between men and women in the ghetto could be described as severely strained during the mid-1960s and through the 1970s. Neither males nor females possessed adequate structural support to function in their ascribed gender roles.

Mainstream role models for motherhood and fatherhood, more prevalent in black neighborhoods in the past, were becoming scarce. Women's roles in connection with motherhood kept a tenuous hold on family stability while male family roles were pushed outside of the decision-making sphere. Women emerged as the economic power holders and males bargained for shares of that bounty with varying degrees of participation in family life. The power scales were tipped once more with the next series of social changes.

LATE-CENTURY CHANGES IN SOCIAL POLICY:
1980S AND 1990S

Citing the decline in marriage and the persistence of the ghetto behaviors described previously, conservative scholars such as Charles
Murray (1984) suggested that ghetto blacks were unsalvageable people because of cultural or genetic deficiencies. The Reagan and Bush
presidential administrations adopted these contentions and created an
atmosphere of political change in which government programs to aid
and train ghetto blacks were eliminated or severely curtailed (Wilson,
1987). Thus, other sources of mainstream connections for poor blacks
were cut off. The final wave of middle and working classes left inner-
city neighborhoods, and the process that Waquant and Wilson (1991)
call "hyper-ghettoization" became complete. Institutions such as
black churches abandoned inner cities with the middle and working
classes. Certainly, some black churches have remained in the inner-
city neighborhoods in which they were founded, but many of these
churches have become *commuter churches.* A commuter church is
one in which the congregation and ministerial staff reside in suburbs
and commute to attend services on Sundays. Monday through Saturday, commuter churches are closed. Few if any of the poor people
who live nearby attend the church. They would not fit in with the
well-dressed, socially conscious churchgoers. Access to religious institutions that once provided help and social roles to poor blacks became limited. The change in the demographics and nature of black
churches is another consequence of the breakup of black communities.

The decline in marriage among inner-city residents is also complete. The institution of marriage has become so uncommon that men
and women rarely view it as a life option and certainly do not connect
marriage to the upbringing of children (Massey and Denton, 1999;
Wilson, 1996). Moreover, the tension between men and women has
risen to open hostility (Massey and Denton, 1999).

Anderson's (1990) monograph *Streetwise: Race, Class, and Change
in an Urban Community* examines the complex relationship between
poor, black young men and women in the inner-city context. Within
the backdrop of economic and social deprivation the goals of young
women and young men are shaped by dim future expectations for
their lives. Sexual conquest without commitment is a primary goal for

men. Achieving commitment from men through sexual favors is the hope of women. Sex has become the sole basis for male-female relationships. The conflicting goals of poor black men and women along with irresponsible sex have had the socially devastating consequence of children born to young, ill-prepared parents with loose connections to each other and without the benefit of a social-support network. Concomitantly, Massey and Denton (1999) suggest that the hostility between poor black men and women is evidenced by lyrics of the late-century, black street cultural symbol, rap music. The lyrics emphasize the conflicting goals suggested by Anderson (1990). Both male and female rappers describe the opposite sex in explicitly sexual and derisive terms and emphasize disappointment and even disgust with male-female relationships (Massey and Denton, 1999). Moreover, their findings suggest that the sexualized images of men and women are internalized completely by both genders. The highly sexual nature of inner-city male-female relationships and gender-generated tension enhanced the potential for the denigration of women in the coming crack cocaine culture.

ANALYSIS OF THE INFLUENCE OF CRACK ON GENDER ROLES

The historical record reveals the metamorphosis of an artificially constructed, isolated, field-slave culture and its artificially constructed gender roles into an isolated sharecropper culture and finally into an isolated ghetto culture. At every step in the transformation, involvement in this culture placed groups of blacks at an extreme disadvantage to those outside the culture and truncated their ability to gain access to the mainstream. It is important to note that the ghetto culture is not a remnant of an ancient cultural heritage of Africa. Neither is it a pattern of genetically inscribed behaviors unique to blacks.

The ghetto culture was formed by the bleak realities of American slavery and the sustained isolation of those farthest removed from the ruling classes. By the 1980s, the safety valves that formerly held the ghetto culture in check by providing access to the dominant culture were essentially gone. The struggles of disadvantaged blacks have been present since slavery. The struggles were first masked by the social organization of the slave system and later by segregation in housing. The concentration of the poor in strictly defined inner-city neighborhoods has brought their problems to the forefront of social science inquiry. Moreover, their plight demonstrates that the devastating experience of slavery has impacted some segments of the black population more deeply than others.

The isolated, inner-city poor neighborhoods have striking parallels with the plantation field hand communities. The plantation field hand communities were isolated from the main plantation house and were characterized by broken families, dependence on others for subsistence, and economically and socially powerless men. Poverty-stricken urban dwellers are often isolated from the mainstream of society and have similar characteristics to the plantation field hands. The development of the urban underclass is the result of a natural progression of events in which the long-term neglect of the poorest subgroups of black Americans has finally surfaced and assumed a geographical dimension.

Working through the history of black women and American racial dynamics, gender roles for black women have been severely circumscribed with overemphasis on sexuality and fecundity. As well, damage to the black male's status in the larger culture put women in the position of balancing traditional feminine roles with roles commonly associated with men—those of family provider for example. It is clear that many black women have been challenged with role conflict, and the evidence in the literature suggests that poverty is a determinant of severe forms of this role conflict. The independence poor black women gained with access to the welfare system has not garnered enough power for them to demand more from the men in their lives. The independence women experienced could be described as symbolic. In the same way that Moore (1969) described the position of ghetto black men as masculinity without status, the position of ghetto black women could be described as femininity without status. Women continue to establish relationships with men who are unable to function adequately in family life and are willing to settle for much less than mainstream ideals. As the discussion on males in the ghetto indicates, men have developed strategies to share economic resources with the women but only minimally share family responsibilities. One could argue that as income decreases, the female role primacy in sustaining poor black families increases and the male role primacy decreases.

The symbolic independence of women has exacerbated the tension with men and created an atmosphere in which violence against women is possible when competition for the scare resources results in favor of the woman. If the women fail to be impressed by whatever strategy the men use to obtain portions of the family income, the threat of violence looms. Men placed in the position of having to negotiate with or manipulate women for resources may feel emasculated by these processes. The men also may feel emasculated by society because of their inability to find life-sustaining work.

Women's power in these communities can be considered marginal, but it is still significant. Women are patently responsible for any family stability among poor blacks. This delicate balance of power changed dramatically with the introduction of crack cocaine. The introduction of crack cocaine to inner cities was the coup de grâce to these disenfranchised and neglected Americans. Crack not only provided many poor black men with a means to obtain income; it provided economic and social power. Crack has provided poor black men with the means to play out fantasies of social power that they have long been denied. The female vulnerability attributable to her sexualized identity has evolved into the site for these power-fantasy plays. The poorest man with as little as ten dollars (sometimes much less) or a crack rock can often demand sex from any crack-using poor black woman. The men can demand the type of sex that they desire and choose the woman who will gratify that desire. This phenomenon extends far beyond the actual sex act. Women who exchange sex for crack are often humiliated by having to perform unspeakable and dangerous acts just to provide a feeling of empowerment to the men. Horrific stories of sadism, gang rapes, and bestiality are pervasive in the sex-for-crack literature. The tense relationship between poor black men and women has intensified and become more hostile. Crack has become an instrument of power in the hands of whoever possesses it and is a powerful, uplifting tool for a disenfranchised male.

Men reclaimed economic and social dominance without strengthening family ties or increasing procreative responsibility. In the past, as described previously, men developed individual strategies for obtaining portions of welfare income. However, these strategies required at least minimal participation in family responsibilities. With the onset of the crack culture men needed only to have crack, and the lion's share of the public assistance could be theirs. It's interesting to note that most of this money is funneled out of poor neighborhoods and into the hands of high-level drug dealers, making the experience of poverty worse for children. Despite their acts of dominance, these men are still dependent on the women for access to the larger society. Apartments in public housing are far more easily obtained by women with children than by single men. Nevertheless, access to these apartments can be obtained by introducing women to crack or by promising large profits for use of the place as a crack house. Crack and its metastatic culture overturned the primacy of females in male-female relationships.

Gender-based sex rules in crack houses also place poor black women in a precarious position. In this environment the sexualized image of black women has been pushed beyond former boundaries and all women in crack houses have been relegated to whore status. By using crack, black women have relinquished any semblance of respectability in their communities.

If job loss is central to the death of black fatherhood among the poor, crack cocaine could be central to the death of black motherhood. Robert Staples (1994) suggests that crack has done more damage to poor black families than did slavery and segregation by destroying the vital link between mother and child and thereby destroying the last vestige of family structure. Losing the ability to care for one's children due to drug use is much more than child neglect for poor black women and their children. Motherhood is crucial for the development of a healthy self-concept and is the basis for family formation. The women lose their only source of self-esteem and identity and the children lose their only source of consistent parenting.

Poor black women of childbearing age who have become involved in crack consumption have opened a huge responsibility gap that the extended family system cannot adequately fill. Social marginalization is doubled for crack-using women. Marginalized by the larger society even before crack, women who use crack become further marginalized within their own smaller communities and become stigmatized as traitors to the venerated status of a black mother. The role of a crack user is antithetical to motherhood.

Black mothers are traditionally described as nurturing, stable, clean, chaste, and providers for the family (Hill Collins, 1994; Stack, 1974). In contrast, the crack-using sex worker is often depicted as selfish, unstable, dirty, promiscuous, and as a money squanderer (Inciardi, 1989; Kearney et al., 1994; Ratner, 1993). Successfully fulfilling the duties, responsibilities, and sacrifices of motherhood endows poor black women with social honor and pride. The functions and attributes of a crack user are a source of shame, embarrassment, and humiliation. The high status role of motherhood is overshadowed by the low status role of a crack user, making women pariahs in their neighborhoods.

The stigma attached to black female crack users points to the gender-based double standard of parental responsibility. Failing to assume paternal responsibility did not accord poor black men social stigma. Indeed, in the black male street-corner culture, flight from responsibility of one's offspring is often revered as "cool." As indicated previously, procreation without long-term commitment to children is taken for granted by many poor black men. In sharp contrast, the experience of female crack users and the subsequent breakdown of caregiving for poor black children is blamed on the women only. The important distinction that should be made at this point is that poor black children had geometrically fewer human and economic resources even before their mothers became addicted to crack by virtue of their biological father's lack of involvement in their upbringing.

As explained in Chapter 1, poor black female crack users who exchange sex for crack rarely use birth control and are not likely to have an abortion when pregnant. Exchanging sex for crack further diminishes the women's gender power from an already low status. More important, pregnancies produced by sex-for-crack exchange further challenge the nature of black motherhood. Although poor black women became accustomed to deteriorating male involvement in family life many years before the crack culture set in and learned to harbor low expectations from men, at least some form of relationship precluded the conception of children. Sex-for-crack conceived pregnancies and the children produced introduced new categories of social and familial relationships.

Conceptions such as these emphasize the woman's vulnerability to the drug and to the male-dominated crack culture. Women who become pregnant by these exchanges may feel trapped due to a culturally constructed aversion to abortion, and may give birth to a child toward whom she may be ambivalent. Caring for a child who may be considered a symbol of her loss of self to drug use may be more than some women can bear. It may be difficult to provide unconditional love to a child bearing this kind of stigma. Guilt may develop as a result of the difficulties associated with parenting a sex-for-crack child. Since pride in parenting is such an important factor for esteem among this demographic group, the role conflict between mothering and using crack is pushed to the limit with sex-for-crack conceptions.

Crack sales, consumption, and sexual acts in exchange for the drug have so dominated inner cities that the addict culture can no longer be considered a subculture. The crack culture is no longer confined to the periphery of the inner-city society; it has become the fabric of the society. The crack economy, social organization, and culture provide inner-city poor blacks with a status hierarchy based on access to the drug along with sets of roles, norms, and values within a tight-knit, inescapable geographic domain. The adherents of mainstream values are now the minority in inner cities.

Crack-related businesses generate the most revenue and provide the most jobs for poor blacks—especially young men. Few people in inner-city neighborhoods are unaffected by crack. The drug dealers who possess material goods and cash are role models for young inner-city men and women. Crack-house proprietors, who are generally older and have relatively stable resources, have become role models as well. The role of the crack addict, although central to the social organization of crack culture, is one of the lowest ranked roles. Unlike other roles in the crack hierarchy, the more an individual takes on the characteristics and expectations of a user the more he or she is derided and thus loses social status. Poor black women were shunted into the lowest ranked roles in the social order and were subjected to a loss of power as men regained control of the income flowing into the community.

The ghetto street culture contained within it elements that helped the decadent gender relations in the crack culture develop. The sexualized markers of femininity and masculinity established during slavery, the strained relationships between men and women, and the estrangement of poor black men from connubial ties opened the door for the unprecedented denigration of black women associated with crack use. Poor black women were very familiar with the male strategies before the introduction of crack to finesse them into having sex or sharing resources. Crack simply provided men with a more direct and mean-spirited way of obtaining money and sex from women. A notable congruency exists between the ghetto culture and the crack culture: both emphasize manipulation of women by men. However, in the crack world the manipulation takes the form of humiliation. Another convergence between the two cultures is revealed in bartering for sex. Men in the ghetto culture sometimes give women token sums of money to have some involvement with the family or for the privilege of having sex. This type of borderline prostitution could be considered a precursor to the exchanging of sex for crack. The similarities between the ghetto and crack cultures partially explain the strong commitment to the crack-user role for some women. Ghetto-related social processes are not completely unlike crack social process. Crack appears to have taken ghetto social interaction to another level of development.

The erratic behaviors and lifestyle of a crack-using woman are contradictory with the stability and consistency required of mothering. For black women, motherhood has historical significance, and up until the crack epidemic was a consistently accessible life status. Although the importance of motherhood for poor black women remains high, involvement with crack lessens the ability to successfully function in a mothering capacity. Losing children to foster care or family intervention is a common occurrence for women users. Loss of this integral part of one's identity serves to perpetuate and increase drug use. This may lead to increasing procreative risk taking and result in additional pregnancies in order to hold on to the status of motherhood. If the drug use continues, the process starts over again, with removal of the child from custody or worse—neglect of the child.

The crack culture exerts a strong force on women users to keep using, regardless of whether they are pregnant or have children. Resisting the crack compulsion is confounded by the structure of the culture itself. Sex-for-crack pregnancies add another dimension to the complexities of mothering while addicted to crack. Pregnancies occurring in this way are paradoxical. The pregnancy is a symbol of the mother's drug use, and at the same time, pregnancy for poor black women is symbolic of their personal identities. For individual women this could mean giving birth to the inopportune child if the identification with motherhood can be achieved. On the other hand, if the woman's identity is firmly invested in the role of crack user, she may choose to abort the pregnancy.

Poor black women are not strangers to role conflict. Most experienced this phenomenon before using crack. Conflicts and paradoxes are characteristics of life for black women, regardless of socioeconomic status. Their life experiences are always shadowed by white mainstream standards for womanhood, which are difficult to realize for women of any race. Black women in general have found methods for defining *self* independent of the larger culture's imposing criteria, but the poor women are more structurally constrained by limits on their educational opportunities, by having fewer sources of income, and by their association with a large pool of unmarriageable men. These constraints make balancing multiple responsibilities more likely and coping with them more difficult. For poor black women, raising families alone was thrust upon them by the incremental withdrawal of men from the burden of parenting. In the past thirty years, male disengagement from their offspring escalated and reached a zenith in the 1980s. Crack and its culture of self-gratification gave females the mechanisms to disengage from responsibilities, if only for a few minutes at a time.

Chapter 3

The Crack Culture and Its Roles: The Complexities of Crack Prostitution

The crack culture emerged within a sociocultural system that developed parallel to mainstream sociocultural systems. The inner-city sociocultural system is a result of long-term processes and social interaction patterns that date back to the institution of slavery.

There are four components to understanding poor black women's lives in the crack culture. First, poor black women are structurally constrained in their social roles. The number and availability of mainstream social roles is severely limited for inner-city poor women. Lack of education and marketable skills precludes acquisition of successful career roles. Furthermore, the unbalanced sex ratio and high mortality and incarnation rates among black men preclude spousal roles for men and women (Darity and Myers, 1992; Jackson, 1971). In addition, disorganized communities with limited resources preclude community-involvement roles (Wilson, 1996). Marginal economic resources in isolated inner-city neighborhoods place further limitations on participation in cultural and civic activities within the larger sphere as well.

Second, although constrained by economic and social factors, poor black women in the crack culture can and do negotiate and enact roles for themselves dependent upon personalities, temperament, and circumstances. Third, female sex in poor black communities in general and particularly in the crack culture comes with sets of expectations and limitations that are difficult to overcome. Fourth, the history and complexities of life as a black person in the American hegemony is also framed with a set of constraints and gender expectations that undergird power relationships in the crack culture.

ADDICT'S ROLES

Stephens (1991) developed an integrated role as structure/role as process theory of heroin addiction based on findings from a number of ethnographic studies. His treatise explains the experience of heroin use. Among other findings, he enumerated a series of research premises concerning the street-addict role and tested them with findings from ethnographic studies conducted by himself and others.

According to Stephens (1991),

> There is a subculture of street addicts. Within this subculture, a master (or central) role exists, the components of which are organized about the expected use of heroin . . . This master role is highly valued by members of the subculture, and the more one's behavior approximates the role, the higher one's status is in the subculture. The street addict role provides meaningful social and personal rewards to those who play it. There are a number of secondary roles in the subculture which are organized around the master role of street addict. These other roles (such as dealer, tout, steerer, etc.) function to maintain the subculture, especially the status of the master role. (p. 42)

Furthermore, the members of the heroin subculture are described as "antisocial" individuals who trust few people and eschew middle-class values. They have almost no friends outside of the subculture and maintain emotional distance with their in-group associates. Impression management is very important to them. When not pursuing drugs, the quest for cash, cars, and clothes generally consumes much of their time. Stephens (1991) also argues that street addicts seldom make long-range plans and prefer immediate gratification of personal needs. A highly valued skill among this group is the ability to con and manipulate others into providing them with money, sex, drugs, or whatever else the addict desires at a particular moment. Being "cool" is also an important impression to make among peers. The aforementioned qualities give the addict social acceptance and status within the group. The "good person," or someone with middle-class values (work ethic, sobriety, etc.) are deviant in street-addict culture.

In addition, Stephens (1991) argues that commitment to the addict role is associated with greater heroin use, and that the commitment is "the degree of investment which a person has both in a certain image of his or her self and in the enactment of certain roles through interaction with others. The more committed a person is to a certain identity or role, the higher the salience of that role" (Stephens, 1991, p. 42). He argues that role commitment will be strong for individuals who have significant interaction with the addict subculture. If social roles before the onset of drug use overlap with components of the street-addict role, the "cool" persona for example, the probability is higher that an individual will be socialized into the street-addict role. Stephens (1991) suggests that role conflict that "occurs when the behaviors demanded by one role are contradictory or inconsistent with the demands of another role" (pp. 59-60) is associated with attempts to become abstinent. Moreover, his classic example of role conflict is the dilemma faced by addicted mothers. The fast-paced lifestyle of the addict and the responsibilities of motherhood are so opposed to each other that many women break down and seek treatment (Stephens, 1991).

Stephens' (1991) description of the street-addict subculture bears striking parallels to two cultures long associated with inner-city life: the culture-of-poverty subculture (Lewis, 1965) and the black male street-corner culture (Anderson, 1978; Hannerz, 1969). Here again, the close relationship between structural conditions and individual behaviors is evident.

The culture-of-poverty subculture is described as a pathological social-organization pattern characterized by family disorganization, substance abuse, inadequate child-rearing practices, the quest for immediate gratification of shortsighted goals, impulsive behavior, crime, and myriad other unfavorable stereotypes. Oscar Lewis's (1965) original study concerned Latin Americans. However, the thesis is commonly applied to urban poor blacks. The black male street-corner culture has been the subject of a number of ethnographies (Anderson, 1978; Hannerz, 1969; Liebow, 1967). The men who participate in this lifestyle are endowed with similar qualities and project the same "cool" images as Stephen's (1991) heroin users. It's arguable whether the street-addict culture developed out of the culture-of-poverty subculture or vice versa. It is difficult to determine which of the subcultures flourished first, but, to be sure, a synthesis has occurred in the wake of the crack cocaine phenomenon in inner cities.

THE CRACK CULTURE

The subcultures of poverty and the black male street-corner culture have become completely dominated by the crack cocaine culture. Whereas deviant subcultures such as those associated with poverty had remained on the periphery of the social organization, the crack cocaine culture has become pervasive in inner-city environments. Crack production, sales, consumption, and associated social structures have changed the landscape of inner cities. After its introduction, crack distribution quickly filled the job vacuum created by late-century economic upheavals so much that men, women, and even children began to occupy roles related to crack production, sales, or consumption. Inner-city neighborhoods have literally become crack manufacturing and distribution machines. Cottage industries have developed around crack consumption and the crack-related sex industry. In the early 1980s, crack was cooked up by mom-and-pop entrepreneurs in inner-city kitchens. At the beginning of the crack era, these base houses contained the manufacturing elements, distribution and packaging components, user amenities, and some had brothel-like atmospheres as well. Base houses were the predecessors of crack houses.

Roles in base houses developed that involved the preparation of the cocaine powder into the precipitate "crack" rock. One role is the "cooker," or the individual responsible for applying the heat source to the cocaine and the other ingredients that form crack. This requires skill and is a high status role in the drug culture. Others are responsible for weighing and measuring the input and the output in this process (Sterk-Elifson and Elifson, 1993). These high status roles have become more infrequent as the means of production has become more centralized and removed from the experience of actual drug use (Maher and Daly, 1996).

When enormous profits were made, organized crime factions moved into the inner city and created crack corporations (Witkin, 1991). The structure of drug trafficking changed so that small manufacturers were squeezed out and the market became dominated by intricate networks of distribution led by drug kingpins. Gordon Witkin's (1991) exposé on the creation of the crack economy sheds light on the development of additional roles and recruitment strategies in the emerging, highly structured crack machines:

Organization brought structure—CEOs, lieutenants, distributors, lab operators, runners, enforcers, and street dealers. The business even went high tech as telephone beepers became tools of the trade. Finding the workers for these groups wasn't difficult. Many inner city teens felt shut off from legitimate economic opportunity and came to see drug dealing as the only path to prosperity. Workers were easily recruited to distribute the drug, but the power structure shifted upward. The glass ceiling effect created by the centralization of control of crack production helped to spread the drug across the country. Since local crack dealers could only advance to a point in the production hierarchy, they increased profits by introducing the drug to other cities. (Witkin, 1991, pp. 44-53)

As the structure of the drug traffic changed and as more individuals entered the crack business, most crack houses become confined to sales, consumption, and sex (Inciardi et al., 1993).

Other roles have also developed in the crack economy. There are distributors at all income levels, "look-out" personnel who watch for the police, and "catchers" who move the drugs quickly in the event of a police raid (Williams, 1989). Crack houses are commonplace in inner cities.

CRACK HOUSES

In the 1980s the crack-house industry blossomed in inner cities all over the country (Inciardi et al., 1993; Ratner, 1993; Williams, 1989). These establishments began because people wanted a private place to cook crack and smoke it. However, as the manufacturing and distribution of crack became more centralized and as more people became involved with either selling or using crack, crack houses became distribution centers and quasi-brothels.

A crack house can originate in any number of ways, take any structural form, and provide any combination of services ranging from selling, purchasing, or smoking crack, and seeking or selling sex. They can start in anyone's house or apartment or spontaneously develop as people congregate in an abandoned building.

A number of ethnographic studies have presented crack-house typologies (Geter, 1994; Inciardi, 1995; Inciardi and Surratt, 2001).

Geter (1994) distinguishes four types of crack houses in Philadelphia based on the socioeconomic status of the proprietor and customers, control of the activities therein, and the state of the facility. For example, a semiprivate, well-kept "party house" is operated by a female addict who supports her drug habit by allowing her home to be used as a haven for employed, working-class men to use crack and purchase sexual favors. The proprietor screens both customers and sex workers for suitability and activities in the house are held in check by the proprietor. At the other end of the spectrum is a "bandominium" (abandoned house/condominium). This unlivable facility, typically an abandoned building or apartment, is a haven for the most desperate users and predatory criminals. Anything can happen in these crack houses; there is no one in control of activities. In the early to mid-1980s, local television news shows frequently reported raids on crack houses in cities all over the country.

In 1986, the "crack house" law was passed and became a component of United States Code regarding illegal drug offences. Statute 21 USC 846 subjects owners, managers, lessees, agents, employees, and mortgagees of any place for the purpose of manufacturing, distributing, or using controlled substances to criminal penalties of up to twenty years imprisonment and fines up to $500,000. However, this legislation did not deter the development of crack dens. Inciardi and Surratt (2001) report that by the late 1990s in Miami the more raucous and bold public crack houses, characterized by violence and debauchery, had disappeared in favor of more clandestine locations in private residences.

The important issues concerning crack houses are (1) that anyone with an apartment or residence can start a crack house; (2) they are chaotic, dangerous places even under the best of circumstances; and (3) great amounts of money change hands. Crack houses are money-making opportunities. Literally everything in crack houses is for sale. Addicts in search of a place to smoke or have sex must pay entrance fees, purchase crack, pay to smoke or use drug paraphernalia, pay for sexual favors, pay for the room to have sex, and in some cases pay for the mattress used for sex (Inciardi, 1995; Inciardi and Surratt, 2001; Inciardi et al., 1993; Ratner, 1993). The profit motive drives the crack house industry. No matter how much money a patron has previously spent in a crack house, when his or her supply of cash is depleted, any courtesy extended to him or her vanishes. Crack house proprietors do not allow people who are not actively purchasing goods or services to remain in the house. Likewise, if a crack whore is not actively taking care of customers or preparing to take care of customers, she cannot remain in the house. There are specific roles that have developed and rules that apply in crack houses that people in the crack world understand.

CRACK HOUSE ROLES AND RULES

Crack houses have organizational structures and distinct roles for people who run the houses, smoke in the houses, or purchase drugs or have sex there. A high-level dealer can set up a house in an abandoned building or apartment and confine activities to drug sales only. A resident in public housing can start a house by simply allowing others to come in and smoke, for a fee. A male dealer can establish a relationship with a woman in public housing and set up a house in her apartment allowing sales, smoking, and sex in specified rooms. These are just a few examples. When word spreads that a place to smoke or purchase crack is available, users appear. Usually one man, or less often a woman, is in charge of all activities in the crack house. This individual oversees smoking, designates rooms for sex, and is in charge of selling the drugs. To enter a crack house, a cover charge of cash or a house hit (a single dose of crack) must be paid to the proprietor of the house. Some proprietors will allow only access to their facilities to people they know to discourage entrance to undercover police and other undesirables such as freeloaders. Other proprietors open their doors to anyone with cash or drugs. The rules of the crack house are understood by all. A woman who shares a man's crack supply is obliged to perform a sexual act in exchange for smoking. Men who smoke with other men are not required to do so. This phenomenon is a clear example of gender bias and is exemplary of male primacy in the crack culture.

Similar to the role of heroin addict, the role of crack user involves specific expectations, self-presentation, and patterns of behavior that distinguish participants. These behaviors include proficiency with use of drug paraphernalia, familiarity with smoking techniques and jargon, and being a member of "the crowd." Cocaine has been demonstrated to be a social drug, rarely used by a lone participant. People are initiated into drug use by friends, family, and associates (Waldorf et al., 1991). There are specific settings for crack use, for example crack houses or at a special "friend's" house or apartment.

In contrast with the user in heroin culture, the user in crack culture occupies a low status role. Although the user is the bread and butter of the economy without whom the other components of the network would collapse, crack consumers are not treated as valued customers (Bourgois, 1989). This may be connected to gender bias due to the number of addicted women or may be because of the behaviors associated with crack use. Crack users are expected to behave strangely. Names in the culture have emerged to label the phenomenon, for example *geek, geek monster, rock star,* and *zombie.* The very short crack high is followed by a dramatic crash or immediate lowering of mood. The craving for the experience sets in again quickly. The user is driven to look for more crack or to get more money to buy the drug, generally in a wild-eyed frenzy. The intense craving for crack makes it difficult to control or limit use. Binging for days at a time until the body literally collapses from exhaustion is very common (Inciardi et al., 1993; Ratner, 1993). Sometimes compulsive foraging behavior occurs (Rosse et al., 1993). Foraging for crack on the floor, furniture, or other places, in search of any small piece of the drug is a sure sign that a user has become a "geek monster." Paranoia is also common among crack users. Many cannot control the urge to look out of a window or cover windows for fear of others looking in (Inciardi et al., 1993).

Users often attempt to assume other roles in the network, for example, becoming a dealer to support the habit, but an addicted individual is usually not successful at other roles due to their use of the drug. Since the roles that involve preparation and sales of crack need a market for their product, inner-city neighborhoods are pressured by these individuals to use crack. Friends will often entice friends to use (Anderson, 1990). The support for the crack-user role in inner-city poor areas is great. However, users do not have the power as consumers to drive prices down or demand better treatment or quality of the product from the distributors.

As with the role of the heroin addict, the role of crack user fills the gaps in life devoid of meaningful activity created by chronic unemployment and loose social alliances. In the initial stages, assuming the role of a crack user is a social phenomenon shared with associates or is a personal response to a life crisis. However, after addiction, the crack use becomes a compulsion that provides time-consuming activity and distracts the individual from anything except immediate reality. Rosenbaum (1981) has discussed the beginning phase of heroin use for women, which serves as a guide for crack use as well. She reports that when learning to use heroin, the processes of *copping* (acquiring the drug) and *hustling* (panhandling or pandering) can be very exciting to the neophyte user. Crack users experience the same kind of excitement. At first, many people try the drug with a friend, relative, or love interest. Learning how to inhale the smoke produced by burning the crack rocks takes a certain amount of skill. After discovering the euphoria of the crack high, the user must then discover where and how to purchase the drug. In the inner city, locating crack is not difficult. Most of the time a trip to the apartment next door or house down the street is all that is necessary. After copping, users learn to prepare the crack rocks for smoking by cutting larger portions into individual doses. They also learn to use a variety of methods of smoking the drug. Ready-made glass crack pipes and "straight shooters" (glass tubes) may be purchased at enabling neighborhood convenience stores. The aforementioned paraphernalia can be costly and take away from the user's supply of drug money. Inventive users may construct makeshift crack pipes from empty beverage cans or plastic aspirin bottles. When the crack compulsion fully emerges the user must find a way to support the drug habit on a daily basis. Usually, household possessions are targeted for liquidation first.

If the user has a VCR, television, a boom box (radio, audiotape, or compact disc player), or any other appliance that can be easily carried out of their dwelling places, these are the first to go. Personal items such as watches and jewelry are easily traded for drugs as well (Bourgois, 1989). After all of the users' possessions have gone up in smoke, they may approach the dealer to whom they gave all of their worldly goods with the hope that he or she will appreciate the user's loyalty extended to him or her. However, the dealer will generally suggest a quid-pro-quo alternative: I will give you this for that. In the case of a male dealer, for men the favor may mean running an errand or relaying a message to another dealer (Williams, 1989), but for most women this arrangement requires that a sexual favor must be provided to the dealer or to one of his drug customers. Here again the gender bias is apparent. The sexual acts represent the power relationship. The dealer who possesses crack has the power to demand sex from women and they usually comply. The crack user and the sex worker are used, abused, and disrespected by those who sell them crack (Fullilove et al., 1992). Regardless of the amount of money an individual has given to a dealer or spent in a crack house, when that user is out of money, possessions, or unable to provide another sexual act, that person is either shunned or thrown out of the crack house.

The crack culture is self-centered, profit-driven, and unforgiving. This attitude starts at the top of the social hierarchy and filters down to the users at the bottom. Users also harbor contempt for other users, prostitution clients, and the drug dealers. Users sometimes develop relationships with people who have money or drugs in order to share their supply. When the drugs and money are exhausted, the relationship is over. That user will then go in search of someone else with drugs or money. Crack-using women practice this strategy more than men.

THE ROLE OF BLACK WOMEN IN THE CRACK CULTURE

Roles for women users in general are limited to a narrow range in the crack world. Few black women are involved in high-level drug dealing, and then usually through association with men. Concomitantly, white or Hispanic women are much more likely to be involved in the upper tiers of the crack-distribution hierarchy. The roles are fewer, more truncated, and more problematic for poor black female users. Roles for poor black women are confined to very-low-level independent dealing, crack house facilitation for others, running a crack house for oneself, or crack prostitution.

First, dabbling at very-low-level dealing is one option for the black female crack user. Some women maximize the return from purchasing crack by obtaining more than they plan to use and selling the balance at a slightly inflated price. For example, a woman may purchase two large crack rocks for forty dollars and convert one rock into two and sell those for twenty dollars each. She gets her initial investment back and has a large rock to smoke as well. Many outsiders, such as suburban users cruising inner-city neighborhoods for drugs, may not realize the size value of rocks and will pay twenty dollars for a rock worth only ten. Women use this to their advantage.

Second, running crack houses for others is a common pattern for inner-city women, especially those who reside in public housing. Women who have an apartment lease or access to other housing have become very attractive to dealers. This is another situation in which an engendered power relationship exists. Some dealers establish a relationship with a woman in order to set up a crack business in her apartment. Enormous profits with minimal effort and minimal household disruption are promised, but rarely realized.

Maher and Daly (1996) argue that any woman with an apartment in the inner-city environment is vulnerable to having her living place commandeered by drug dealers and used for crack distribution and consumption. The following statement from one of their research participants, a forty-year-old black woman in inner-city New York, is an example of how women with access to housing can be exploited.

> I started selling crack. From my house. (For who?) Some Jamaican. (How did you get hooked up with that?) Through my boyfriend. . . . They were supposed to pay me something like $150 a week rent, then something off the profits. They used to . . . like not give me the money. . . . I went through a whole lot of different dealers. Eventually, I stopped payin' the rent because I wanted to get a transfer out of there, to get away from everything 'cause soon as one group of crack dealers would get out, another group would come along. (So how long did that go on for?) About four years. Then I lost my apartment, and I sat out in the street. (Maher and Daly, 1996, p. 479)

Once the door was opened, the woman could not stop the flood of dealers into her home. She had to take drastic measures to stop it. The dealers had the option of setting up business in another woman's apartment; she had none. This woman ended up homeless.

A third option for poor black women is running an independent crack-consumption place in her home. Some women support their habits by allowing others to smoke crack in their homes. Occasionally these entrepreneurs will rent rooms for "guests" to engage in sexual activities or introduce male guests to girlfriends who will provide sex for crack or cash. These arrangements are generally short lived; low-level crack houses of this type are easy for law enforcement to bust (Maher and Daly, 1996). They present much less danger than higher level crack houses run by Uzi-toting men.

The fourth option, by far the most common role for poor black women in the crack economy, is that of the sex worker. There are real differences between street crack sex workers and live-in, crack-house sex workers. Women who become street workers usually have a place to stay and a support structure outside of the crack world, no matter how weak, in place. Women who live in crack houses are dependent on the crack dealer for life's necessities and have little if any autonomy.

The role of the crack street ho (whore) requires learning a specific set of skills. Presentation of self figures heavily in this equation. The crack craving and competition on the streets compels many women to wear very provocative and often revealing clothing. Hair and nail grooming is essential. Braving traffic is hazardous and much skill is required in flagging down approaching vehicles containing potential clientele. These women learn how to spot potential clients who cruise the neighborhoods looking for cheap, fast sex. Furthermore, they learn to make split-second evaluations of potential sex customers. The wrong decision could mean a jail sentence if the solicitor is an undercover police officer. The sex worker could also become the victim of violence or perhaps risk death with a less-than-accurate evaluation of a customer. Crack sex workers are known to be less particular and are willing to take more risks than heroin users in the selection of clients (Inciardi et al., 1993).

Geographical areas, referred to as the "ho strolls," or the known cruising streets, are learned by the street workers. They know the hotels, boarding houses, and other areas in which sex can take place. Crack house proprietors are frequently amenable to "working girls" who bring their "dates" to crack houses. Rooms can be rented by the half hour for fees of five to ten dollars plus entrance charge (Inciardi et al., 1993). This arrangement can be beneficial to all, especially if the "date" purchases more crack when there. Crack sex workers also master the art of hastening the sex act, the art of the deal, and the artful dodge of law enforcement officers. Some even defend themselves against men who may refuse to pay after an act is accomplished by getting the money first. The more the crack compulsion dominates the woman's life the more desperate she becomes for the drug and thus willing to abandon all of the aforementioned skills, hygiene habits, and safety precautions (Ratner, 1993; Inciardi et al., 1993).

Crack house sex workers who live in crack houses are not as independent as street workers and are subject to more abuse and degradation than freelance prostitutes. Their role is to provide sex to crack house customers. They are not always paid for their services. A crack house proprietor may extend a woman's services to a purchaser of a large amount of crack as a "freebie." When residential sex workers are paid, the amount is often very low, frequently that of the lowest value for a hit of crack ($3) or simply for a smoke (Inciardi et al., 1993). The heavy traffic in crack houses and twenty-four-hour activity make privacy difficult. Clearly this is a lifestyle of desperation.

Little is known about women and girls who live in crack houses. Most ethnographic accounts center on the experience of street walkers (Inciardi, 1989; Inciaridi et al., 1993; Maher and Daly, 1996; Ratner, 1993) or women in treatment or other institutional settings (Beaty-Muller and Boyle, 1996; Fullilove et al., 1992; Miller, 1995; Pursley-Crotteau and Stern, 1996). Women on the street, in treatment centers, or in jail are easier to access and interview.

James Inciardi and colleagues' 1993 monograph on women and crack cocaine use contains the following description of the life of a crack house girl that provides revealing information.

> Upon entering a room in the rear of the crack house (what I later learned was called a freak room), I observed what appeared to be the gang-rape of an unconscious child. Emaciated, seemingly comatose, and likely no older than 14 or 15 years of age, she was lying spread-eagled on a filthy mattress while four men in succession had vaginal intercourse with her. After they had finished and left the room, however, it became clear that, because of her age, it was indeed rape, but it had not been forcible rape in the legal sense of the term. She opened her eyes and looked about to see if anyone was waiting. When she realized that our purpose there was not for sex, she wiped her groin with a ragged beach towel, covered herself with half of a tattered sheet (affecting a somewhat peculiar sense of modesty), and rolled over in an attempt to sleep. Almost immediately, she was disturbed by the door man, who brought a customer to her for oral sex. He just walked up to her with an erect penis in his hand, said nothing to her, and she proceeded to oblige him . . . the dealer/informant explained that she was a "house girl"—a person in the employ of the crack house owner. He gave her food, a place to sleep, and all the crack she wanted; in return, she provided sex—any type

and amount of sex—to his crack house customers. (Inciardi
et al., 1993, p. 154)

The preceding situation may be an extreme example or may be the
definitive experience. The life of females who live under these conditions is an area in need of further study. There are many unanswered
questions about their lives. How do these girls come to such an arrangement? Could these girls who have grown up in the crack houses
know no other lifestyle? Whatever the answers, females who live in
crack houses are among the most ravaged by the culture and are
clearly sexual minions of crack house proprietors.

Women are at an extreme disadvantage in the crack world and are
disproportionately channeled into the lowest roles, even under the
best circumstances. They have varying degrees of success in other
roles, but the role women can count on consistently is that of a crack
prostitute. The greater participation of poor women in general and
poor black women in particular in crack-related sex has undermined
the social stability for the impoverished. Women as sex objects is in-
tegrally woven into the fabric of the crack culture. This view makes it
difficult for women to be taken seriously enough to occupy other,
more powerful roles in the social structure. The potential for sex is always a looming possibility for women crack users who interact with
men. Increases in prostitution among poor black women has contributed to exacerbating the stereotype of women as sex objects. The historic stereotyping of black women as highly sexual beings and the
traditional gender role parameters predisposed them for subordina-
tion. Problematic gender role development in the male hegemony has
long been associated with poor black women. Elwood and colleagues
(1997) stress the economic powerlessness of poor black women that
places them at risk for exchanging sex for crack cocaine, and they point
to the centrality of gender roles for poor black women. The combination of few resources and a strong gender role identification creates a
power deficit for black women in the male dominated crack culture.

CRACK ROLES VERSUS GENDER ROLES

Rodney Stark stresses that "gender roles are not the only roles that
influence self-conception. Occupation, hobbies, education, marital
status—all influence how we see ourselves. But none has as much in-

fluence as do our gender roles" (Stark, 1994, p. 168). Gender roles are especially important for inner-city poor black women because other social roles (for example, community leader), career roles, and so on, are generally limited.

A number of scholars have described the structure of poor black families as matriarchies with women assuming the role of stable breadwinner due to the relative ease with which females function successfully within the dominant society (Bernard, 1966; Frazier, 1939; Moore, 1969; Moynihan, 1965; Rainwater, 1970; Stack, 1974). Gender roles commonly associated with poor black women are mother, female head of household, and extended family leader. These pivotal roles are among the few choices available to marginalized women as a source of status and life satisfaction. Black family literature in particular highlights the importance of the historical role of mother as a stabilizing force and conduit for socialization (Frazier, 1939; Guttman, 1976; Bernard, 1966; Staples, 1991a,c). Conversely, the roles of men in the family context are frequently characterized as intermittent, secondary, and dependent upon women (Bernard, 1966; Hannerz, 1969; Liebow, 1967; Moore, 1969). Moore (1969) specifically describes the role of poor black men as "masculinity without status." He argues that since few options are available to achieve success in a career, these men retreat from family responsibility and take pride in functioning as a sire of offspring. The economic marginality, frustration with the role of provider, and retreat from parental responsibility are frequently occurring themes concerning the roles of poor black men.

The introduction of crack cocaine to poor black communities in the mid-1980s has resulted in a dramatic shift in the balance of power for women and men with devastating results for entire families. Crack cocaine use initially negatively impacted motherhood through intrauterine drug consumption (Bateman et al., 1993), and later through child neglect and abuse. More than fifteen years following its appearance in inner-city neighborhoods, crack use has damaged the role of female head of household by draining public assistance resources (Minkler and Roe, 1993; Staples, 1991c). The high rate of crack use is associated with a rise in homelessness among the urban poor. In some cases, crack cocaine has dismantled or weakened the extended family system that once served as a safety net against the systemic barriers that deter economic and social success within the dominant culture (Staples, 1991c). Furthermore, crack has empowered some marginalized men within the crack cocaine underground economy (Williams, 1989). These individuals had few economic opportunities before the drug's introduction, and have surfaced as controlling agents in the crack culture. The evidence suggests that a role reversal has occurred (McCoy et al., 1996). Many women in these communities, who have already suffered from the effects of societal rejection find their situation worsened as a result of crack use (Anderson, 1990; Fullilove et al., 1992).

Motherhood and supporting roles within extended family networks are among those available for poor black women that are sanctioned by society. Motherhood is often prescribed for women in this context. The opposing schools of thought concerning poverty and black families highlight the importance of the mother among poor black families. The "culture of poverty" theorists (Moynihan, 1965; Murray, 1984) and the "adaptive strategy" theorists (Anderson, 1978; Billingsley, 1968, 1992; Hannerz, 1969; Hatchett and Jackson, 1993; Liebow, 1967; Moore, 1969; Rainwater, 1970; Stack, 1974; Staples, 1971, 1978, 1986, 1991a, 1994; Sudarkasa, 1993) agree that the poor black population overwhelmingly consists of mothers and their children. They also agree that motherhood is central to family formation. The culture-of-poverty theorists contend that family composition of this type is pathological and due to inherent or derived cultural deficits. Conversely, the adaptive-strategy theorists argue that the female-headed household family pattern is a survival tactic and a creative cultural adaptation to an oppressive social and economic system, and that is a natural response to the lack of breadwinner jobs for many poor black men.

Motherhood has been a source of status and life satisfaction for impoverished black women since slavery. As mentioned before, black family literature in particular highlights the importance of the mother as a stabilizing force and conduit for socialization (Bernard, 1966; Frazier, 1939; Guttman, 1976; Staples, 1991a).

The disparity between the high status role of motherhood and the low status role of sex worker suggests role conflict. Patricia Hill Collins (1991, 1994), suggests that motherhood in black culture is a symbol of power, a source of family stability, and a focal point for community organization. The meaning of motherhood is thus challenged by women who exchange sex for crack. The roles associated with sex worker are characterized by a prevailing desperation for crack (Ratner, 1993). Having exhausted other means of supporting the habit, the body becomes the marketable commodity. The degradation that these women face and the subsequent devaluation of women's roles is antithetical to the traditional image of motherhood in black—especially poor black—communities (Fullilove et al., 1992). Black mothers are traditionally described as nurturing, stable, clean, chaste, and as providers for the family (Hill Collins, 1994; Stack, 1974). In contrast, the crack sex worker is often depicted as selfish, unstable, dirty, promiscuous, and as a money squanderer (Inciardi, 1989; Kearney et al., 1994; Ratner, 1993). The disparity between these roles offers opportunities for the development of unique life adaptations and survival mechanisms that suggest processes of role enactment.

As mentioned earlier, crack use and motherhood are often polar opposites in terms of role performance. In addition, the role of mother and the role of crack user both demand a significant investment of time and energy. Crack-using mothers often use creative strategies for balancing crack-use role performance and mother role performance (Kearney et al., 1994a). Since the two roles cannot coexist, they must compete for time, resulting in one status overshadowing the other.

GENDER RELATIONSHIPS
IN THE CRACK CULTURE

Gender relationships figure heavily into the crack social structure. The crack culture is gender biased, with men dominating the social terrain. The gender dynamics described in Chapter 2 are central to understanding the sex-for-crack phenomenon. Sexualized images of black males and females, structural constraints on the earning power of black men, and female role primacy in black families created the conditions for a shift in the balance of power between men and women in the poor black communities.

In the past, women's access to income transfers gave them economic power. Access to crack confers power and control to the men who had been economically powerless in the larger society. Sex as a site for the expression of power and dominance undergirds the entire crack culture (Beaty-Muller and Boyle, 1996; Henderson et al., 1994; Miller, 1995). The crack literature is saturated with distressing accounts of unimaginable, degrading, and sadistic sexual acts demanded of women who exchange sex for crack (Inciaridi et al., 1993; Ratner, 1993). The horrific descriptions do not bear repeating here. Suffice it to say that some men in control of crack cocaine behave as cruel directors in the theater of the absurd orgies that occur in crack houses and other crack-consumption places. Many men are attracted to the events in crack houses that endow them with the masculine dominance denied to them by the larger culture (Bourgios, 1996). Consider this quote from McCoy and colleagues (1996):

> The prostitution of the past . . . has been replaced by orgies called "wild thangs" in which women exchange sex for "rocks" (pieces of crack). One sex party host explained: "You'd just better not take that first smoke . . . because the men watch you and see how you react and when you want more they control you, they can do anything." . . . Another choreographer of sex parties explained . . . [t]he "party" held in this room, begins with three women who he has lured with an offer of a free first "hit" of crack . . . if they want another hit, they must strip down to their undergarments. By the third hit, they are at the mercy of the host. (p. 89)

Men who possess crack have the power to orchestrate the actions of the women with whom they smoke. As demonstrated in the previous example, as the compulsive crack smoking escalates, the humiliation of women escalates. The man's feeling of power and domination increases accordingly. Prostitution, then, in the crack culture, is embedded in the struggle for masculine authority among disenfranchised black males.

DEFINING SEX-FOR-CRACK EXCHANGE

Prostitution as a means to support a drug habit is not unique. Female heroin users have historically supported their addiction with sex for money (Rosenbaum, 1981; Sterk, 1990; Stephens, 1991). Some, however, termed the "bag brides," actually exchanged sex for bags of heroin (Goldstein, 1979). The literature on sex-for-crack exchange, based on ethnographic and other studies all over the United States, have remarkably similar findings. The leitmotiv in all of these studies is a combination of degradation, devaluation of human life, domination and humiliation of others, and violence (Fullilove et al., 1993; Inciardi, 1989; Inciardi et al., 1993; Muller and Boyle, 1996; Ratner, 1993). Women who exchange sex for crack occupy the bottom tier of the crack social organization.

Exchanging sex for drugs rather than money is unique in the crack culture in that heroin and other drug users prefer to exchange sex for money. The money may be used to purchase drugs, but receiving money for sex is considered a step above receiving drugs, and it gives a sense of control to the user (Inciardi et al., 1993).

Mitchell Ratner's ground breaking study *Crack Pipe As Pimp* (1993) defines sex for crack as exchanging sexual acts for the drug itself or exchanging sex for the money to buy crack. Furthermore, he developed a typology that differentiates three types of sex for crack exchanges: (1) casual, (2) sex for money for crack, and (3) sex for crack. Casual exchanges are infrequent, opportunistic transactions that occur in social settings and sometimes in bars. These types of exchanges may occur with men the women may know only casually, but with whom they have sexual encounters. The second type of exchange, sex for money for crack, is distinguished by the type of woman (or man) engaged in the prostitution, the separation of crack consumption from the actual act of prostitution, and the preference for money rather than the drug itself. Prostitutes who also use crack (as opposed to crack users who prostitute themselves) engage in these types of exchanges. Ratner (1993) stresses as well that the compulsiveness of the crack-use cycle is the distinguishing marker that separates these exchanges from simple prostitution. The third type of exchange, sex for crack, is the lowest form of exchange, and is controlled less by the prostitute and more by the customer. The woman (or man) is desperate for crack and will engage in sex for the smallest unit value of crack or the dollar equivalent. This can be as low as two or three dollars, and sometimes less. Women who engage in sex for crack are denigrated within the crack culture. They are termed "hos" and "skeezers" and a variety of other pejorative names (Fullilove et al., 1992; Mahan, 1996). Their bodies are literally reduced to a sum total of parts that can be used for a variety of perverse sexual acts for little more than a hit of crack cocaine.

James Inciardi and colleagues (1993), make distinctions between sex for crack on the street and sex for crack in crack houses. They also distinguish between professional prostitutes who use crack and crack addicts who support their habits with prostitution. The women and sometimes men who make their living as street sex workers are often able to exercise more control over the selection of partners, the price for services, the acts they perform, and the degree of exposure to health or other risks. Professional prostitutes prefer and in some cases demand money for services rendered as opposed to drugs. The money may be later used to purchase drugs, but the prostitute makes the decision. Conversely, crack house sex is entirely controlled by the proprietor of the house. Usually a man, this person sets the prices, designates which rooms may be used for sex, and generally oversees all activities, sexual or otherwise, that occur in the house. The male customers select the woman they wish to have sex with and demand the service they desire as well. Crack house girls/women have little control over what happens to them. They are characterized as much more desperate for the drug than street workers.

Crack houses have implicit rules that vary from house to house, but in general the people who possess the drug have and exercise power over those who do not. Men have more access to money and crack, so they dominate women in crack houses. Women who smoke in crack houses understand that smoking with a man often requires a sex act in exchange with no negotiation of price or type of sexual act performed. The man who possesses the crack gets what he desires. In this setting, Inciardi and colleagues (1993) further distinguish between girls/women who live in crack houses and girls/women who visit these houses to use drugs. Girls/women who simply visit these houses to smoke have the option of leaving if the situation becomes too unbearable. The girls/women who live in the house are not as fortunate. Usually they are younger, sometimes very young teenagers, and are homeless, abandoned, and have no place to go.

The crack house proprietor provides them with a place to live, food, and drugs in exchange for providing sexual services to customers in the house. These girls/women must perform any sex act until the customer is satisfied. Satisfaction may be extremely difficult if the man is a chronic crack user. Prolonged crack use makes maintaining a penile erection and achieving orgasm an arduous task (Inciardi et al., 1993).

This book uses Ratner's (1993) definition of sex for crack described previously. Sex for money to purchase crack has become such a fundamental part of the drug-support process for significant numbers of women that the long-term results are the same as exchanging sex directly for the drug. The money is converted to crack so quickly after each sexual act is completed that the possibility of other uses for the money has become remote. Thus, the second and third types of exchanges in his typology have become blurred in very recent years. Women often exchange sex for crack and/or money, dependent on day-to-day circumstances; however, for most, the money is so quickly spent on crack that any measured spending of funds is precluded.

The studies on sex-for-crack exchange agree that crack-related prostitution has cheapened the price of sex, increased the potential for violence, and put women who engage in this behavior at a severe disadvantage (Elwood et al., 1997; Forney et al., 1992; Fullilove et al., 1992; Goldstein et al., 1992; Inciardi, 1989; Inciardi et al., 1993; Miller, 1995; Ratner, 1993). Eventually, most women who use crack, regardless of where they fit in the aforementioned sex-for-crack continuum, hit bottom. The crack compulsion will ultimately drive the sex-negotiation process for street walkers and subject crack house sex workers to lengthy, degrading acts for very little drug in return. Although Ratner's (1993) study was comprised of aggregated data extracted from major cities all over the United States and Inciardi's (1993) study was conducted in Miami, Florida, similarities were discovered among women as crack encroached upon Atlanta. Many of the same issues were common to the women in the present study.

Chapter 4

A Picture of the Women

IDENTIFICATION OF THE WOMEN STUDIED

Fifty-two poor black female crack users were formally screened with the screening instrument. The screening instrument, a brief, two-page, coded questionnaire that could be administered in five minutes or less, was used to ascertain whether women exchanged sex for crack, how often they exchanged sex for crack, whether they contracted sexually transmitted diseases, their HIV positive or negative status, and if they had ever become pregnant by exchanging sex for crack. The frequency and outcomes of sex-for-crack pregnancies were recorded also. The instrument included demographic information as well, for example, highest education level reached and income earned at legal jobs.

Of the forty-six women who exchanged sex for crack, twenty-three women reported one or more sex-for-crack pregnancies. Women who became pregnant were asked to participate in a longer, in-depth, audiotaped interview. Among twenty-three eligible women, nineteen in-depth interviews were completed.

The quantitative data are reported for the crack users screened (52), and used to compare women who exchanged sex for crack (46) with those who did not (6), and used to compare women who became pregnant (23) with those who did not (23). Table 4.1 compares the two groups on selected demographic variables.

The six female crack users who reported not exchanging sex for crack were not included in the remainder of the analysis. Five of the women were middle-aged (ages 39, 42, 45, 45, and 47) and one was age 21. Their mean age worked out to 39.83 with a standard deviation of 9.64. Three of these women completed high school. One completed the tenth grade and the other two the eleventh grade, with a mean education of grade level 11.33 and standard deviation of .82.

TABLE 4.1. Demographic characteristics of women who exchange sex for crack and women who do not exchange sex for crack.

Characteristic	Women who exchange (N = 46)	Women who do not (N = 6)
Age (in years)	34.57 (± 6.03)	39.83 (± 9.64)
	[18-47]	[21-47]
Education (in years)	10.96 (± 1.81)	11.33 (± .82)
	[7-16]	[10-12]
Income (estimated dollars per year at a legal job)	< 5,000 [44]	< 5,000 [5]
	<10,000 [2]	<10,000 [1]
Crack-use frequency (in days per week)	5.89 (± 1.80)	6.00 (± 1.67)
	[1-7]	[3-7]
Sex-for-crack exchange frequency (in days per week)	4.15 (± 2.39)	—
	(0-7)[a]	
HIV results	HIV+ 7	HIV+ 3
	HIV– 37[b]	HIV– 3

[a]Three women exchanged sex for crack less than once per week. Their sex-for-crack frequencies were scored "0."
[b]Two women were not tested for HIV infection.

One woman reported earning more than $5,000 but less than $10,000 per year at a legitimate job and the other five earned less than $5,000 per year. Although they reported not exchanging sex for crack, they reported using crack frequently. The range of days per week of crack use for this small group was 3 to 7 days per week, with a mean of 6.0 and standard deviation of 1.67. All of them had been tested for HIV infection and three of them reported an HIV-positive status. As a final note about the women in this group, t-tests were executed to identify differences between those who exchanged sex for crack and those who did not on the following factors: income ($t = -1.2/p = .23$), education ($t = .499/p = .62$), age ($t = 1.87/p = .067$), HIV-positive status ($t = 1.7/p = .082$). No significant differences were found. The results for both age and HIV-positive status showed the greatest difference. The small sample size precludes more meaningful interpretation of these statistics.

WOMEN WHO EXCHANGED SEX FOR CRACK

The range of ages for the women who exchange sex for crack ($N = 46$) was 18 to 47. The mean age was computed to 34.57 with a standard deviation of 6.03. Highest education completed ranged from seventh grade to college and computed to a mean of 10.96 with a standard deviation of 1.81. Interestingly, education levels were split between twenty women who had completed high school or higher and twenty-six women who had an eleventh grade education or lower. Ten women reported completing the eleventh grade, six women finished the tenth grade, five women completed the ninth grade, four women completed the eighth grade, and one woman finished her seventh year of schooling.

Forty-four women reported earning less than $5,000 per year at a legitimate job and two women reported earning more than $5,000 but less than $10,000. Similar to the previously described group, this group reported using crack nearly every day. Mean number of days of crack use per week worked out to 5.89 with a standard deviation of 1.80 (see Table 4.1). Furthermore, thirty of the women reported using crack cocaine daily. The mean number of days per week reported for exchanging sex for crack was 4.15 with a standard deviation of 2.39. Three women reported exchanging sex for crack slightly less than once per week. These three women were included in the study because they had become pregnant at least once in a sex-for-crack exchange. Their sex-for-crack frequency was scored "0," thus the range for exchanging crack was 0 to 7 days per week. Thirty-seven women who exchanged sex for crack reported that they were HIV negative, seven were HIV positive, and two women had not been tested.

Forty-one of the women reported multiple incidences of an array of sexually transmitted diseases including syphilis, gonorrhea, herpes, genital warts, chlamydia, pelvic inflammatory disease, and trichomoniasis. Only five women had never contracted a sexually transmitted disease. Twenty-two of the women used birth control inconsistently while exchanging sex for crack and twenty-four neglected to use any form of birth control or protection. Thirty women identified prostitution as their main means of habit support. The other sixteen reported theft, shoplifting, conning, or obtaining money from friends or relatives as their means of habit support. However, all had engaged in some form of prostitution to continue crack use.

SEX-FOR-CRACK PREGNANCIES
AND THEIR OUTCOMES

Within the sample of forty-six women who exchanged sex for crack cocaine at least once per week, twenty-three women reported the incidence of one or more sex-for-crack conceived pregnancies in their reproductive histories. Table 4.2 presents a comparison of demographic data for the women who became pregnant by exchange and those who avoided sex-for-crack pregnancies. There were very slight differences in age and education between women who became pregnant and those who did not. The mean age for those who became pregnant was 33.30 with a standard deviation of 6.64, and the mean age of those who had not become pregnant was 35.83 with a standard deviation of 5.18. Mean education for those reporting sex-for-crack pregnancies was 10.70 years with a standard deviation of 2.10. For those who had not become pregnant by sex for crack exchange the mean was 11.22 with a standard deviation of 1.48. Results of the t-test analysis showed that these minor differences were probably due to chance in the following categories: age ($t = 1.43/p = .15$) and educa-

TABLE 4.2. Demographic characteristics of women who became pregnant by sex for crack and those who did not.

Characteristic	Pregnant by exchange ($n = 23$)	Not pregnant by exchange ($n = 23$)
Age (in years)	33.30 (± 6.64)	35.83 (± 5.18)
	[18-47]	[27-44]
Education (in years)	10.70 (± 2.10)	11.22 (± 1.48)
	[7-16]	[8-14]
Income (estimated dollars per year at a legal job)	< 5,000 [22]	< 5,000 [22]
	< 10,000 [1]	< 10,000 [1]
Crack-use frequency (in days per week)	6.43 (± 1.24)	5.35 (± 2.12)
	[3-7]	[1-7]
Sex-for-crack exchange frequency (in days per week)	4.74 (± 2.24)	3.57 (± 2.45)
HIV results	HIV+ 2	HIV+ 5
	HIV− 20+[a]	HIV− 17[a]

[a]Two women were not tested for HIV infection.

tion (t = .975/p = .33). Among those who had not become pregnant, five out of the twenty-three were HIV positive, and in the pregnancy group, two out of the twenty-three were HIV positive.

A majority of women who had become pregnant engaged in high-volume crack use. The mean number of days per week of crack use was 6.43 with a standard deviation of 1.24. Eighteen women in the pregnancy group reported daily crack consumption. The range of crack frequency for this group was three to seven days per week. These women exchanged sex for crack more often than those who did not become pregnant. Mean sex-for-crack frequency computed to 4.74 days per week with a standard deviation of 2.24. Twenty women exchanged sex for crack three times per week or more, with ten of the twenty reporting daily sex-for-crack exchanges.

Eleven of the women reported that they became pregnant more than once due to sex-for-crack exchanges. Five had become pregnant twice, five had become pregnant three times, and one woman had become pregnant four times. A total of forty-one pregnancies were reported. Seven pregnancies were terminated by elective abortion, seven were terminated by spontaneous abortion, three were tubal pregnancies, two resulted in stillbirths, seventeen resulted in live births, and five women were pregnant at the time of contact with the intent to deliver (see Table 4.3). Abortions were chosen by three women only. Two of them had three aborted sex-for-crack pregnancies and the other had one such abortion. Interestingly, the women who chose to have abortions were not similar in terms of education level. One woman received several years of education beyond high school, another had completed eleventh grade, and the other had completed tenth grade only.

Table 4.4 presents a comparison of birth-control use of the pregnant and nonpregnant groups. Sixteen out of the twenty-three women who became pregnant by exchange did not use any form of birth control during sex-for-crack encounters. The remaining seven designated condoms as their primary means of preventing pregnancies, though use was inconsistent. This will be discussed more fully in the next section. The nonpregnant group reported using condoms (ten), birth control pills (one), injections (one), or had had their fallopian tubes tied (three) to prevent pregnancies. However, eight women in this group reported using nothing at all to prevent sexually transmitted diseases or pregnancy while engaging in sex-for-crack transactions.

TABLE 4.3. Sex-for-crack pregnancy outcomes.

Outcome	Frequency	Percent	Cumulative percent
Live births	17	41.5	41.5
Pregnant now	5	12.2	53.7
Stillbirths	2	4.9	58.5
Tubal pregnancies	3	7.3	65.9
Miscarriages	7	17.1	82.9
Abortions	7	17.1	100.0
Total	41		

TABLE 4.4. Birth control methods for pregnant/nonpregnant groups.

Birth control method	Pregnant group	Nonpregnant group
Condom	7	10
Pills	0	1
Injections	0	1
Tubes tied	0	3
Nothing	16	8
Total	23	23

WOMEN WHO BECAME PREGNANT

The twenty-three women who became pregnant via sex-for-crack exchange made up the theoretical sample for the ethnographic part of the study. Nineteen of these women were interviewed with the in-depth, semistructured instrument previously described. Four women who became pregnant this way were not available for the in-depth interview. Three disappeared in the underground drug scene before interviews could be completed. Qualitative data was obtained from one of these women before she disappeared. She participated in a focus group conducted during the formative phase of the research. One woman refused to be interviewed. The stories that emerged from the focus group and completed interviews revealed that complex and troubled lives existed well before the onset of crack use. In Chapter 5 the women reveal in their own words how the social and economic forces described in Chapter 1 impacted their lives. Their stories show a pattern of race, class, and gender marginalization along with stressful lives since childhood that support the historical patterns of gender role ambiguity and stereotyping described in Chapter 2. The women describe unstable circumstances into which they were born and report how poverty, truncated education opportunities, parents' substance abuse, limited access to jobs, and disappointing relationships with men ushered them into cycles of personal loss. Analysis of the qualitative data obtained in the in-depth interviews revealed alarmingly similar patterns of experiences and themes. Presentation of the qualitative data will take the form of quotes from women who best represent the common experience of all in the study. We will hear the voices of (pseudonyms) April, Amy, Chaka, Cybil, Danielle, Dena, Kathy, Linda, Sylvia, Toni, and Valerie, whose experiences exemplify poor black women's lives in poverty and in crack addiction. The women describe as well how the introduction of crack cocaine dramatically changed their neighborhoods, their lives, and the lives of their families. When each woman's story is introduced for the first time, her pseudonym appears in bold and is accompanied by a biographical sketch.

Chapter 5

Lives of Women Who Exchange Sex for Crack

Life before crack was far less than ideal for the women who participated in the in-depth interviews. The social and economic forces that shaped the life chances and opportunity structure for poor black people (outlined in Chapter 1) were clearly evident. The combined influences of race, class, and gender marginalization imposed structural constraints on the women's lives and social roles long before the onset of crack use. Lack of family stability appears to be a major force in the lives of nearly all women interviewed.

STRESSED LIFE SITUATIONS

Traumatic childhood experiences and hard-pressed family lives were common to every woman in this part of the study. Beginning in childhood, most of the women drifted from one difficult life situation to the next. Stressed life situations were apparent in a number of different areas: (1) unstable home lives and parents' substance abuse, (2) truncated educational opportunities, (3) limited access to jobs, and (4) unstable relationships with men. These experiences ushered the women into early cycles of personal loss, grief, and the frustrating effects of failure and severely limited access to all except the most fundamental social roles.

Unstable Home Lives and Parents' Substance Abuse

Confusing and unstable home lives along with substance abuse by parents figures heavily in charting the women in the study on destructive life courses. Most of the women were born into poverty-stricken, weak, unstable homes with marginal father participation and in many cases marginal mother participation. Early in these women's lives, instability and fluid family composition, uncertainty, and traumatic experiences were taken for granted as just a part of growing up. Although eleven reported that their parents were legally married, few families remained intact.

Seven women's parents were never married and one woman did not know if her parents had been married. Only four women were raised by both parents. Furthermore, only five women were raised by their biological mothers. Ten women were raised by another relative or by a nonrelative. Figuring heavily in being raised by someone other than a parent was their mother's teenage pregnancy.

Most women recalled few details regarding their families of origin. Many did not know how their families came to live in the Atlanta area and had limited knowledge of their parents' or grandparents' history. Some were uncertain about additional brothers and sisters produced by their fathers. Families with both parents were plagued by other elements consistent with structural poverty, for example, involvement with illegal activities or with substance abuse. In some cases substance abuse by one parent or by both played a critical role in family disruption, the early death of a parent, or in influencing the women's own drug use.

Other family members were involved in substance abuse as well. All nineteen women reported that some members of their families used alcohol or drugs. Brothers, sisters, aunts, uncles, and cousins were described as drug users, and crack was the most frequently mentioned drug.

Truncated Educational Opportunities

Another difficulty experienced by most women in the ethnographic sample was that of obtaining an education. Only four women had completed high school or better. Six women received eleven years of education, three women received ten years of education, and six women received nine years of education or less. Women who dropped out of school were asked why they dropped out of school. Pregnancy was by far the most common response. Eight women became pregnant at some point during their school years and eventually stopped going to classes. Teenage pregnancy is one of the leading causes of poor educational outcomes, poverty, and poor educational outcomes for the children of the adolescent mothers. In addition, offspring of teen mothers have an increased risk of becoming parents during adolescence themselves (Kaplan et al., 2001). Substance abuse also interfered with attaining an education for some women in the study.

Three women cited drug use as the reason for discontinuing their education. Two women stressed the influence of their peers as a contributing factor, and two women cited family or other problems as the reason for leaving school.

Limited Access to Jobs

The combined influence of race, class, and gender marginalization was also evident in the examination of the work histories of the women. The types of legal occupations in which all of the women were employed could be described as low-skill or no-skill professions. These types of jobs—cooking preparation, housekeeping, maintenance work, factory packing, chicken processing, and janitorial work—are traditionally and stereotypically associated with poor black women. Fourteen of the women stated that they held jobs in low-skill professions and four women stated that they held jobs in no-skill professions. One woman had never held a legitimate job. Even those women with high school educations and above reported employment in dead-end, low-paying jobs. All nineteen women had been welfare recipients at some point in their lives.

Unstable Relationships with Men

All of the women described themselves as heterosexual. Only one woman reported a lesbian experience, which was not consensual. The women were forced to perform for their crack while a man watched them. Most women expressed a desire for marriage and a stable family life but felt powerless to achieve these mainstream hallmarks. Furthermore, most reported dissatisfaction and frustration with their relationships with men. Four women out of nineteen had been married. Only two were legally married at the time of the interview, and neither were living with their husband. About half (nine) of the women had very early sexual relationships that produced children. Most of the women recounted having long-term relationships with several men over the course of their lives. These relationships lasted from one and one half years to nine years. Only one woman reported having no long-term relationships with men. This woman stated that her longest relationship lasted only two months. Another woman was a self-described "player" who "just hung out and partied," although she did have a relationship with a man that lasted six years and resulted in one child.

In addition to knowing little about the families into which they were born, a number of the women knew surprisingly little about the men in their lives. For example, when asked how many years of school their partners completed or even their partner's exact ages, many women did not know the answers or they guessed. Some of their partners were drug users. The relationships were frequently based on mutual drug use. Some of their relationships were with drug dealers and were based purely on exchanging sex for drugs.

DIFFICULT BEGINNINGS: LIVES BEFORE CRACK

All of the women were asked about their lives before becoming addicted to crack. Most of them had few life-sustaining or self-defining roles other than those associated with motherhood. As indicated earlier, career opportunities for these women were limited. Opportunities for other sources of life satisfaction, such as involvement in community organizations, were constrained as well. Moreover, most had a tenuous grasp on motherhood related to early, out-of-wedlock pregnancy and the transfer of their children's care to others.

Consider the early experiences of Kathy, Amy, and Dena (not their actual names). Their backgrounds show a pattern of the difficulties mentioned in the previous section. Their experiences are typical of many poor black female crack users. The backgrounds and lives of Kathy, Amy, and Dena are similar to the stories I heard over and over again in this study and in previous studies. Barrier after barrier occurred in their lives that prevented any access to the milestones of mainstream success.

Kathy was thirty-six when interviewed. She went as far as the eighth grade in school. Kathy reported receiving a monthly welfare check of $253. She supplemented her income with an undisclosed amount from prostitution. Her parents were not legally married. She knew the identity of her father but did not know much about him nor did she have a relationship with him. Her mother's profession was reported to be domestic work. Very early in her childhood they lived in public housing. However, her mother had an alcohol addiction that resulted in her premature death, after which the maternal grandmother raised the children. Kathy explains:

My brothers, all us got different daddies. I have two brothers by my mom. I don't know if I have any brothers or sisters by my dad. . . . I lived with my grandmother. She raised us. . . . My mother was an alcoholic. My father was an alcoholic. They just hooked up and had babies, made me or whatever.

At age twelve Kathy found her mother's body, eyes open, on the kitchen floor. Before her mother's death Kathy was responsible for helping her grandmother care for her ailing mother. This situation is severely traumatic to a young girl. Being the oldest child and the only girl in the family, she had to help her grandmother care for her two younger brothers after her mother died. She cites her mother's death as the reason she dropped out of school. Kathy gives more information about why she dropped out of school.

I lost interest [in school] after I woke up one morning and found my mama in the kitchen dead with her eyes open. She was an alcoholic. I had watched after her after she had open heart surgery. They told us that there was nothing they could do for her after the surgery. She came home. She had done swolle[n] up real big. She couldn't get around and I had to see about her. That night, I was laying on the floor; I couldn't sleep. She looked at me. Then she went in my little brothers' room and looked at them, like she knowed that she was fin' to die. She came back and said, "I want you to promise me that you will take care of your brothers." I said, "Yes ma'am." I was twelve. I dozed back off. The next thing I knew, my grandmother woke me up about five o' clock in the morning and said help me get your mama back in the bed. I knew she was dead, her eyes were open and she was looking up at the ceiling. After that, I just gave up. It took something out of me. I loved school. I was good in school, good in math. I was bringing home good report cards. Ever since then I been beating myself up. After the years, I wanted to learn to read because I started having children. But I just couldn't get it. . . . I recall that before she had this open heart surgery. She stayed sick a lot. She couldn't even bathe herself.

A significant portion of Kathy's childhood was lost due to her mother's alcoholism and death. She took on family roles beyond her level of maturity, which cost her an education. She finished the eighth grade only and self-reported that she could not read. Obviously some other constraints were present if she managed to make it to the eighth grade without learning to read. Her lack of education and poor reading skills limited her choices for employment. Kathy reported working at very low-skill jobs, for example, housekeeping at office buildings, hotels, and at a warehouse. She was legally married at age seventeen, but was long separated from her abusive husband at the time of the interview. Kathy reported that her husband introduced her to crack and that he raped her routinely. Even after they had separated, if he saw her on the street, he would pick her up, take her somewhere, and rape her. Kathy explains:

My husband would rape me all the time. . . . He would get violent and twist my arm behind my back or pull me by the hair. Make me go to his house and takes it by force. Whenever he wanted some sex with me, he would catch me walking and demands it.

Kathy has six children, ages two to nineteen. The three older children are her husband's biological offspring. Her older children were in the care of her very elderly grandmother, the children's greatgrandmother. The three youngest resulted from sex-for-crack pregnancies. Her first sex-for-crack pregnancy resulted in the birth of a girl, age seven at the time. The identity of the child's father was not known. Kathy's aunt had custody. Her second sex-for-crack child, a six-year-old girl, was being cared for by her aunt as well. This child's father was also unknown. Kathy's third sex-for-crack child was a two-year-old girl. Her father was unknown as well, but the child was claimed by Kathy's sometime boyfriend. The last child was the only child in her custody.

Amy, twenty-six years old when interviewed, had completed the seventh grade. Though she earned less than $5,000 per year at a legitimate job, she reported earning up to $7,000 per month from prostitution. Amy's alcoholic mother had given her two children up for adoption. She expressed much disappointment in her mother. She also felt shame because she did not know the identity of her father.

I never lived with my mother. . . . My mother is a stoned alcoholic. . . . She gave me and my brother up for adoption when I was an arm baby. I lived in foster homes. . . . I don't know who my father is. . . . I lived with a series of families.

Amy was very articulate and intelligent despite dropping out of school at such a young age. Her difficult home life was not supportive of finishing school. Amy shares why she dropped out:

I completed up to the seventh grade. I was living in a [home for girls]. I was about fourteen [years old]. One of the house mothers there suggested that I was too old to be in that grade and that because I was an obese student that I could get my GED and it was just like a high school diploma. I took her advice. I did that. I took the test and I missed it by one point and I never went back. . . . I was too old. I was easily influenced. That's how I remember. I didn't have a problem going to school and doing my homework. I had gotten left back a couple of times so I was too old to be in that grade. I was having all kinds of problems with my classmates. They upset me. The kids were teasing me about the color of my teeth, my weight, and I was already in a girls' home. It was too much for me.

Most children experience teasing in school. Overweight children are especially targeted for cruel taunts and unflattering remarks. For Amy this sad fact of life could not be buffered by the equalizing effects of a supportive family. A stable home life with nurturing parents could have helped Amy put the name-calling into perspective. Her life spiraled downward as she was shuffled from foster homes to group homes and back to foster homes. She was sexually abused at age six in one of the homes and eventually ran away at age thirteen. She was not on the street long before she met a pimp who introduced her to prostitution. Her first sexual experience was with a paid client. Amy is the woman who reported having no long-term relationships with men. Amy longed to get married, have children, and live in a nice home of her own.

After years of professional prostituting she eventually became addicted to crack. A female friend suggested that she try crack to ease the emotional pain after being rejected by her alcoholic mother again. When she ran out of money for drugs, her experience with prostitution was called into play. Eventually, she shifted to trading sex for crack. Amy reported using condoms with paid customers every time before she started using crack. After she began using crack she started having unprotected sex. Six years later she became pregnant by an unknown client. Amy was seven months pregnant with this child, a boy, when interviewed. This was her first pregnancy. She was devastated because, similar to her mother, she would not be able to share the identity of the father with her child. Amy had a very limited work history. She stated that she had only two short-term jobs: one in a dry-cleaning business and the other as a cook in a day care center.

Dena was twenty-six years old at the time of the interview. She reported earning $2,000 per month with prostitution. Dena's early life was difficult as well. She finished the ninth grade in school and dropped out in the tenth grade due to her pregnancy. Her home life was extremely strained. Dena was the product of an out-of-wedlock teenage pregnancy. Her mother gave birth to Dena at the age of fifteen. Her parents never married. Dena was raised by her maternal grandmother. When Dena was six years of age, she was molested by her "stepdaddy."

My stepdaddy molested me at age six. He only did that once. He harassed me. I didn't give him an opportunity [to do it again]. I lived with my grandmother. I used to go to my mother's house to see my sister. He did it over there. My grandmother found out and I didn't go over there again.

Dena's life became more strained when her grandmother died. Shortly after going to live with her mother at age fifteen, Dena became pregnant. Her mother insisted that she have an abortion. Their relationship deteriorated, and a year later Dena became pregnant again and gave birth to a son. She moved in with a boyfriend when she was seventeen and it was there she was introduced to crack. Dena applied for welfare for her son and used the money instead to purchase crack. Her mother intervened on her grandson's behalf and took custody of the child and charge of the public assistance funds. Dena was not much of a talker. Her interview responses were very brief, but the meaning was always clear.

I was getting my first welfare check, I smoked [crack] it up. My mother said "uh-uh" [no]. My mom was taking care of him. So I signed custody over [to her mother] and she is getting it [welfare for the son].

Her crack habit pushed her in and out of her mother's good graces and her home. At age seventeen Dena's crack compulsion became more intense. Desperate for the drug euphoria and without funds to achieve it, she tried prostitution for the first time. She became pregnant by her first customer.

I never did this [prostitution] before I used crack. I was seventeen when I first did it. I wanted some drugs. That's when I got pregnant with my second child. I was having sex with him for the drugs. I was over [at] my uncle's house. He [a man] told me that he had some money and he would give it to me and I wanted some dope.

This pregnancy pushed Dena over the edge with her mother. Her mother did not come to the hospital to see her new grandchild. Eventually her mother relented and took custody of the baby. However, she asked Dena to move out. Dena went on to have two more sex-for-crack pregnancies. She gave birth to the second sex-for-crack child and again her mother accepted the child into her home. Dena was pregnant with her third sex-for-crack child at the time of the interview.

Dena had a very short work history. She worked as a cashier in 1989 and cleaned an office building, once. She had never been married and reported having only one long-term relationship—with the man who introduced her to crack. Her two other relationships were with much older men. These arrangements were purely for economic resources and shelter.

The lives of Kathy, Amy, and Dena show that even before crack came to inner-city neighborhoods, life was hard for many poverty-stricken young black girls growing up. Their lives are similar to those of the other women in this study. Structural conditions in poor black communities made stable social-role development nearly impossible. The constant barrage of family problems dissolved childhood innocence and interrupted formal learning opportunities. Furthermore, parental shortcomings, especially those of their mothers, set a pattern for motherhood that would be repeated when the women had children of their own. The loss of childhood, the sense of deprivation associated with that loss, and the pattern established by their mothers of shifting the responsibility of child rearing to the previous generation shaped expectations for their adult lives, before and after crack. These expectations would play a dominant role in overwhelming the traditional extended family system.

Even before crack's introduction, the quality of life among poor blacks was sufficiently eroded so that families were broken, schooling was cut short, jobs were limited, and relationships were fragile. Conditions worsened after drug dealers focused on distributing crack cocaine to poor neighborhoods.

THE CRACK TRANSFORMATION

Neighborhood Changes

The women estimated that crack appeared in their neighborhoods as early as 1981 and as late as 1989. Crack filtered down into the South from the North. Some women related that in the mid-eighties they began to see plastic vials of crack in their neighborhoods. Many remembered the early days when people cooked cocaine powder into "free-base." Several women reported knowing how to cook the powder into the solid form. The range of ages for first crack use was 15 to 33 years, with a mean of 22.32 and a standard deviation of 5.83. Three women tried crack for the first time when they were older than age 30.

At first, it was an endless party with friends, neighbors, and relatives, everyone getting high together and having a good time. One of my respondents, Toni, witnessed the early days of crack's introduction to her neighborhood. **Toni,** age twenty-seven, finished the twelfth grade and stated that she earned about $2,400 per month from prostitution. She had never been married. Toni's life was complex. It was difficult to distinguish her boyfriends from her prostitution clients. She established quasi-relationships with some of her "tricks" and had relationships with drug dealers, which resulted in her three sex-for-crack pregnancies. Each pregnancy was brought to term.

Her first sex-for-crack pregnancy resulted in the birth of a boy, age six at the time, whom she gave up for adoption. Her second pregnancy, also a boy, was intended for the same adoptive home but died shortly after birth. The third sex-for-crack pregnancy resulted in the birth of a girl, age three at the time, who was being cared for by her maternal grandmother. Toni had a total of six children. Only four were living. She had one other child die four months after birth. Toni describes how she first became aware of crack:

My cousin had come from Ohio. This was when they were using the little crack vials. Before crack really hit. . . . But they had starting bringing these crack vials from up North. I remember them basing. I saw these great big bowls. They were all in the kitchen just smoking. I kept wondering why my baby['s] daddy kept hanging down there. 'Cause he was young, too. I wanted to know what was really going on. Just about everybody in the neighborhood was in my cousin's apartment. My curiosity got the best of me. So I went into the kitchen with everybody else. 'Cause I saw this cloud going on and these big bowls full of smoke. And everybody was looking "Zombified." Then my cousin said, "Try this." I was the only one who was not addicted.

Partying with crack was very different from the parties in the 1970s during which alcohol and marijuana were consumed. Crack was much more than a mood-altering substance and icebreaker at parties. Crack was a means to make money. As more and more people became involved, the women in the study watched in awe and horror as crack transformed their neighborhoods into drug sales and consumption machines. Strangers in search of drugs began to appear. Organized gangs of dealers encroached on the drug users to take advantage of those who wanted to keep the party going. The crack scene turned ugly for several reasons.

First, the dealers began to compete with each other through violent means over distribution rights and turf issues (Anderson, 1990). Second, the crack craving produced paranoia and an urgency among users that drove them to do almost anything to obtain it (Inciardi et al., 1993; Ratner, 1993). Third, formerly powerless and disenfranchised people could obtain instant power by possessing crack (Bourgois, 1989; Elwood et al., 1997). Thus, incidents of abuse and degradation proliferated.

Amy describes what happened in the neighborhood of one of her foster homes:

It was like one day the kids come home from school they could go outside in the front yard and play. Then, all of a sudden, it's not like that anymore. We had to stay locked up in the house. Because people were on every corner. Sometimes it had gotten so bad that the dope boys would be right in front of your door. Not giving you and your family, your mother, your father no kind of respect. And the kids look out the window and see this kind of activity and they think that it's cool.

As competition escalated between groups of dealers, incidents of violence increased. Furthermore, as users began to exhaust their pools of resources, illegal activities proliferated. The neighborhoods began to change demographically as a result. Kathy tells how it occurred where she lived:

Our neighborhood, we had whites on one side of the street and blacks. . . . It was a black and white neighborhood. Very peaceful. Very quiet. After the crack came in, the white peoples moved out. . . . I remember in my neighborhood, they started breaking in the white folks' houses. You see them and they old [white neighbors]. They [drug users] just walk in and the [white] people can be sittin' on they porches. They wanted them a hit [of crack] so bad that they would walk up on the porch and walk on in them folks' houses and come out with what they want and tell them [the white home owner] "Don't move!" just to get high. . . . The children couldn't go out and play no more, it had got just that bad. You had to watch your children. They had to stay in the house and they wanted to know "Why can't I go outside?" 'Cause it is too much activity going on. Drug dealers hanging out and junkies hanging out. It was just too much. So they [children] wasn't allowed to play outside.

Kathy described a neighborhood under siege. This same transformation occurred in countless inner-city neighborhoods nationwide after the introduction of crack. Previously, drug-related violence, crime, and other activities were confined to the certain areas to be avoided, for example, alleys, or they occurred late at night. With crack's introduction the rules for self-protection changed. People could no longer sit on the porch to enjoy the afternoon air and children could no longer safely play in the yard. Fear and paranoia among residents increased so much so that, as Kathy indicates, whites began to move away. More important, more affluent and stable black families began to move out as well. This exodus essentially removed the neighborhood's last links to mainstream social and cultural values. As the stable, working people moved out, standards for behavior changed dramatically.

The behaviors of the people in these neighborhoods began to change. As people used crack more often, their lives and actions began to change. Simple lives became more complex, seemingly overnight. Becoming involved with crack was more than most people bargained for. Toni conveys the changes she observed in her neighborhood:

I remember the first time seeing some of my friends' parents going out. I was so used to seeing them [behave as] high-class and just subtle, homebound people. All of a sudden, you start seeing them [the wives] on the street, hanging out with different men. And seeing the husbands, just around the homes [not working]. . . . Families just break up. I remember some of my friends, including myself, the teenagers, it wasn't about school and fun anymore. It was about sex and sexual activity and just teenagers being out of hand.

As indicated by the previous responses, the crack toll on poor black families was heavy. Nowhere was this more apparent than in the life of **April** and her family. Her family situation was nearly the worst-case scenario attributable to the crack phenomenon. Her entire family became crack users and this set off a series of family tragedies, including deaths from AIDS, child abuse and neglect, and state-ordered removal of all of the minor children in the family.

April's situation was extremely complex. At the time of the interview April was thirty-three years old. She went as far as the ninth grade in school. Her parents had been legally married, and very early in her life her father was a construction worker and her mother was a housekeeper. Unable to make enough money in construction work, her father turned to drug sales to supplement the family income and support their ten children. This was the beginning of the end of this very large and complicated family. Her father introduced crack to everyone in his family.

The family home became a crack house with children under the age of eighteen living there and smoking crack. April explains:

My daddy started it all. He used to sell drugs. I guess somebody encouraged him to smoke it [crack]. He sold crack. I was about nine years old when it [crack selling] started. My daddy put his whole family on crack. Me, my mama, my sister, my brother, my aunt, my uncle, my niece, my nephew, my cousins would all sit at a table and smoke crack. He [father] was smoking and I guess he wanted her [mother] to see how it feel. Then he called us, all of us kids. I was about fifteen [years old when she first tried crack]. . . . Almost all of my relatives use drugs. I have one sister, out of my whole family, that does not use drugs. . . . My mother died. She died smoking crack and drinking. She had a stroke. She was sixty-two years old.

April began raising herself at age thirteen when her parents' drug use escalated. She never held a legal job and was never married. She had six children, ages one-month-old to eighteen. The youngest was conceived by sex for crack. April became pregnant at age fourteen and dropped out of school. She describes her experience:

I finished the ninth grade. . . . I got pregnant. I hung around with the wrong people. My mama and daddy was on drugs, so I was really taking care of myself. I had a little boyfriend and I got pregnant. I stayed sick so much, I wouldn't go [to] the school. . . . I was fourteen [years old] when I first got pregnant. I had the baby.

As the quote indicates, pregnancy was the ultimate reason the woman dropped out, but she obviously had other family problems due to her parents' drug use. April had relationships with three different men, each of which produced children. Her longest relationship lasted for three years.

April's family was haunted by tragedy brought on by everyone's involvement with crack. She relates the horrific incident that resulted in the child welfare system taking all of the children from April and her sisters. April's youngest sister Carrie surrendered her preschool-aged nieces to a man for sex acts in exchange for the money to purchase crack. The man was mentally ill and had full-blown AIDS. April explains:

There is a curse on our family because of crack. My brother died injecting crack. My twin sister had two stillbirths because of crack. . . . It is sick. It's a lot of crazy stuff be going on and I was right in the middle of it. Doing the crazy stuff too. Tricking. Having sex for crack. Going in empty houses and having sex. I don't think that crack scene has change. It ain't changed to me. . . . It has made fools of women, especially black women. It made us careless, don't care. I've never seen women, especially black women not care about their kids, until crack came out. Would sell their kids for crack. My sister sold my nieces for crack. It was so sick. I smoke crack myself, I was the biggest geek monster in town. But I never would have sold no children, no three- and four-year-old for crack. My niece worried me all night long, she said, "Auntie April, my 'coochie' [genital area] hurts." She had had the chicken pox. I said, girl it ain't nothing but the chicken pox down between your legs.

Me, on crack, I wasn't careful enough. I just didn't think to look. If I had looked I would have seen the big bite mark on her vagina. He had bit her. He licked all in her butt. And he had full blown AIDS. She didn't get AIDS. They test her every three months. She [Carrie, April's sister] got away with it the first time. She had fifteen dollars. She bought them [the kids] a little box of chicken and she bought herself a ten-dollar rock. I asked Kesha, she is the three-year-old. She is real smart. She can tell you everything, detail by detail. I asked her where she got the money for the box of chicken. My sister looked at them, said, "You better not tell!" My sister had scared them so bad till they didn't want to tell what was going on. So the next month came out. I had took the kids to the park. She came to get them again. She said, "Where the girls at?" I said, "What girls? What you want with the girls?" She said, "My friend want them." I said, "What your friend want with them teenagers?" I thought she was talking about my daughter and stepsister. She said, "He don't want them, he want Kesha and Annie. I said, "What the hell he want with them babies?" I said, "I'm fin' to go ask him."

She followed me all the way up the street. She said, "April, don't ask him, don't ask him!!" When I got to the house, I said, "Reg, what you want with them babies?" I said, "I ain't gon' do nothing to you. I ain't gon' mess with you or fight you or nothing." He said, "Oh, I'm want to do to them the same thing I did to them last month." I said, "What did you do to them?" He said, "Oh, I ate one and finger fucked the other one." I said, "Hold on one minute."

I went and beeped my other sisters: my twin sister, the little girls' mother, and my stepsister. I took them back up there. I told them I wanted them to hear what this white mother fucker said. I had all my sisters there to hear what he told me. I told him that we wouldn't do nothing to him. Carrie was steady saying, "You better not tell!" Carrie was the one that did it. She is my youngest sister with my mama and daddy. I said, "Reg, tell us what happened. We ain't gon' do nothing to you." He said "Oh, I ate one and finger fucked the other one. Licked them all in the butt." . . . He used to go around paying people ten dollars for their drawers. He would give people five dollars if you call him a bitch or a bastard. It's so crazy around that place over there. He was getting a check and he would borrow money off his check. He didn't do crack; he was a drunk. I believe he didn't have much sense. Then my sister said, "I'm going to ask you one more time." I said, "You don't have to ask him no more." I had a bat in my hand. That's when I hit him. I flipped. Just knowing that he put his mouth. . . . His mouth was purple and green. He was so sick. He was so nasty. His house had this much trash in it. When he told me that she pulled their panties down and held their legs open while he did that, you know. I don't even remember beating him up like I beat him up. . . . The three-year-old said, "Aunt April, that man ain't gon' mess with me no more, is he?" I said, "He ain't gon' mess with you no more." The three-year-old is with DFACS [Department of Family and Children Services] now and the four-year-old is with her grandmother, her daddy's mother.

This wretched situation made the six o'clock news and the newspapers in Atlanta. Carrie, April's sister, was convicted of child abuse and went to jail. The mentally ill man was convicted also. Social welfare case workers went to the home in which these incidents occurred and placed all of the children—April's, Carrie's, and another sister's—in the care of relatives and with foster families. Losing her children sent April on a yearlong crack binge. She ended up homeless, sleeping in an abandoned house. April witnessed the deterioration of the social and family structures because of crack from the closest possible vantage point. She came of age knowing little of any other lifestyle. Children growing up with crack-addicted parents were all too common in her neighborhood. April describes the crack houses in her neighborhood and relates the experience of a young boy she knew who lived in a crack house and witnessed his mother engaging in prostitution.

Every kind [of crack house] there is. Some have women in them. One room they be having sex. Another room they be freaking, like standing on the table, butt naked, dancing. Another room, they be fucking and sucking. Another room, they be smoking. Then, they have kids in the house. My friend name Lisa. This man I told you that died; he had a crack house. He had one hit room. Her son would be laying up there in the bed, he was thirteen, while they were in there having sex and smoking. I used to make him get out. I would say, "Danny, you can't stay in here, you have to get out." He said, "I done seen my mama sucking, fucking, and smoking" . . . I said, "You mean your mama let you see all of this mess?" Most of the time, I was out tricking, and I wasn't there to see her do all of this in front of him. When I got there, he'd be asleep or sitting up in the front room and they steady be smoking. He be trying to watch TV. He'd be hungry. His mother be done geeked up the food stamps and her check. I would buy him something at Church's [chicken]. I would say, "Come on, Danny, I'll get you something to eat." He said, "I sho do appreciate it, April." He said, "You seen my mama?" I said, "Last time I seen her, she was on the ho stroll." . . .

I smoked in empty houses and crack houses. . . . The same house [that she was previously discussing]. One bedroom, a kitchen, and a front room. Most of the time it was dirty. The same house where the little boy was in the bed-room, asleep or in the front room asleep, I had to go the bathroom or to the kitchen to smoke. . . . This was a man friend's house. I smoked with the man that owned the house.

Jane Hansen's (1998a,b,c,d,e) *Atlanta Journal and Constitution* weeklong series titled "Growing Up with Crack" vividly describes the stressed lives of children born to crack-addicted mothers. Her findings were similar if not identical to the findings in this book. From the time these children are born, often drug exposed at birth, they face the trauma of coming home to the chaotic lifestyle of a marginalized woman with few resources to care for a child, and the looming potential that his or her mother's crack habit will take prece-dence over his or her care and well-being.

As explained, some children of crack-addicted mothers are unfor-tunate enough to either live or spend time in crack houses. They are frequently left unsupervised and are often malnourished and are ex-posed to unimaginable acts beyond their level of maturity and com-prehension. Their mother's public-assistance resources are directed away from their care and into financing her drug use. Crack houses are described as dirty and dangerous places, unsuitable for habitation by anyone, let alone children. Even though April engaged in the same activities as Danny's mother, she drew the line when it came to expos-ing her children to her crack habit. She tried her best to make sure her children were cared for by someone else when she was on the "ho stroll." As indicated previously, she also tried to act as a guardian for other crack-addicted women's children in her neighborhood.

April was extremely ashamed of the horrendous events that befell her family. Another one of her sisters, Eliza, died of AIDS. April re-lated that Eliza had three sex-for-crack children, all of whom were in-fected with HIV. April shared that one of these children was dead from the disease and the other two were extremely ill. She was openly hostile toward her father for addicting the entire family. Her father was at the time ill with Alzheimer's disease, high blood pressure, and ulcers, among other things. She reported, "He doesn't even know who he is." She was also embarrassed by her involvement in crack prostitution. Most of the women in the study were ashamed that the crack addiction led to exchanging sexual acts to continue drug use.

As mentioned in Chapter 1, in the mid-1980s, inner-city neighborhoods had reached a critical zenith of economic and social transition. As can be clearly seen from the women's lives, even before the introduction of crack cocaine, many of the families remaining in inner cities were fragile, poor, and struggling with multiple threats to family stability. In addition, as described in Chapter 2, families were held together tenuously as births to teenage mothers pressed responsibility of raising children to previous generations, and male participation in family life diminished. Crack cocaine's appearance into this house of cards pushed the neighborhoods and the families within them over the proverbial cliff and into nearly total estrangement from mainstream American society, and with it, mainstream values. These neighborhoods became dangerous and unhealthy places to live as crack-related crime and sexual activities achieved prominence in everyday life. In addition, with the shortened years between generations attributable to multigenerational teenage pregnancy, two or perhaps three generations of young people have grown up knowing no other lifestyle, other than fantasies seen on television.

Chapter 6 focuses on the process by which the women's quasi-relationships with men evolved into prostitution. Here we find reasons why they engage in sexual risk taking. In addition, the women shared strategies they use, in spite of their relatively low rank in the crack world, to harness some sense of power and control in their lives.

Chapter 6

Exchanging Sex for Crack and Sexual Risk Taking

SEX FOR CRACK INITIATION: TRANSITION FROM QUASI-RELATIONSHIPS TO PROSTITUTION

Many poor black women spend significant portions of their lives alone (Bernard, 1966; Staples, 1994; Wilson, 1987, 1996). The lives of women in the present study clearly support this assertion. Recall that of nineteen women who participated in the ethnographic interviews, only four had been legally married, two of whom were divorced and none of whom were currently living with their husbands.

The shrinking pool of marriageable men coupled with high mortality and incarceration rates for poor black men places poor black women in the unenviable position of being in surplus. Large numbers of never-married, divorced, or separated poor black women in their 20s, 30s, and even 40s are unable to settle down, marry, and move on to other phases of life. Many women are looking for the right man and are constantly disappointed by their relationships. The serial relationship pattern of the women in the present study supports this contention. The women experience a long extension of the adolescent "dating" stage of life. It is within this context that sex-for-crack bartering developed.

Prostitution for crack is not easily understood. When the poor black female crack users in this study perform sexual acts directly for drugs or for the money to purchase drugs they do so with an intricate web of partners. For many, their unstable relationships with men have become more unstable. The age range for first sex-for-crack experience was 17 to 35 years with a mean of 24.26 and standard deviation of 5.91. Five women reported exchanging sex for crack for the first time after the age of 30.

In the early years of the crack phenomenon, sharing crack with men at parties may have led to sex in conjunction with a mutual attraction. The sexual activity in the crack context evolved into a male social expectation and later into a social norm. Some women's relationships with men are now based purely on obtaining crack. Some enter relationships with the hope of commitment from the men with whom they share crack. However, these expectations are more often than not unrealized as the men use the drug as an instrument of control, and the women are reduced to performing sex for the crack they smoke. Some women become involved with dealers in order to get closer to large supplies of crack or were attracted to the money and material goods these dealers could provide. Other women simply use prostitution with strangers on the "ho stroll" or in crack houses as a means to continue getting high on a daily basis. The range of partners and range of situations in which sex for crack occurs are varied. Moreover, any woman in particular may engage in any or all of the sex-for-crack scenarios mentioned previously. Thus, this type of prostitution is not easily equated with basic street prostitution.

Exchanging sex for crack was a unique experience for each woman in this study. However, there were notable differences between the women who had had prostitution experience before becoming addicted and those women who had not. Four out of the nineteen women had engaged in prostitution for money before their addiction to crack. Women with this experience viewed the sex-for-crack phenomenon in a slightly different way than others. Prostitution was entered into as a means of survival for these four women, and thus exchanging sex for crack was just another step, albeit downward, in the quest to stay alive. Amy, who became a street walker at an early age, explains:

It was different for me because I ran away from a foster home and got tangled up with a pimp. A real live pimp. I was about thirteen or fourteen. He introduced me to prostitution. This was before the dope. I hooked up with him. They taught me how to prostitute, to survive. He took care of us. I left him and got hooked up with another pimp. I think I hooked up with about three of them before the police found me. The lady whose foster home I ran away from had a missing person's thing out on me. But I had been through three pimps. That's how I knew that when I ran out of money that I could prostitute and get more money in order to get high. So it started way before [the crack].

Furthermore, women who were ladies of the evening before crack use were likely to use protection while prostituting, but after becoming addicted, acknowledged that crack interfered with self-protection. Again, Amy shares her thoughts on this subject:

When I was whoring professionally, I practiced safe sex. My pimp gave us condoms. And a man couldn't do anything to me if he didn't use a condom, not matter how much money he had. My pimp told me, even if the man had a hundred dollars, he had to use a condom. When I was doing it for crack that's when I didn't practice it [safe sex].

The preceding passage points to the freelance nature of crack prostitution. Crack street prostitutes are generally not supervised or protected by pimps. After she became addicted to crack, Amy moved from the protection of pimps to exchanging sex to support her crack habit and fell into the pattern of not using condoms during sexual acts. Moreover, the self-absorbed, "every man or woman for himself or herself" nature of the crack culture is alluded to by Amy's statements.

Women who were prostitutes before crack also made sharp distinctions between prostitution for money and sex for crack. Amy articulates this in following statement:

The difference is that when you are prostituting, it's like a profession. The men know that you are a prostitute and not a crackhead; they handle you different. They know somewhere in the background there is a man watching to make sure that they don't get out of line with his girl. When they know that you are doing it when you are addicted to dope, you just might wind up getting anything done to you. That's the difference.

Women whose first prostitution experiences were linked to their crack addiction viewed exchanging sex for crack as an act of desperation. Most of these women were baffled and dismayed at the power of the crack addiction to suck them into the sex-trade business. Many at first tried other means to get money, but as their resources dwindled and the crack craving fell upon them, the final showdown emerged. Kathy relates her first sex-for-crack experience:

I didn't believe that I would do it. 'Cause I was married. He [her husband] happened to leave one night and the urge came down, the craving for it. I wanted it and I didn't have no money. The first thing I started doing was looking at my stereo and my VCR. That went first. I starting taking everything out the house before I started turning tricks. Because I was one of the types that said I wouldn't let it get me that bad; I wouldn't go that far. As long as I got some shit [belongings], answering machine, in here. Everything started go-

ing, piece by piece, in the house that had some value. Then I started realiz-
ing that they were taking advantage of me because I didn't get but twenty
dollars and I paid three hundred and some dollars for this TV. So I said that I
would just put it in pawn. So after I had took everything out of the house, by
the next day, here I am broke again. So I had to turn my first trick. I felt so
cheap because I did it for just enough to get me a sack [of crack] with. I felt so
used and so cheap.

First-time prostitution in the context of crack use left the women
with feelings of shame and disgust. This was especially true if the
man did not live up to his end of the bargain. The women related accounts of very often being "ripped off" by clients. For example, a man
might proposition a woman and promise to pay a certain amount in
cash, drugs, or both for a specific type of sex. When the act is completed the man refuses to pay, or rather pays a portion of the promised
amount. This was a common experience for crack prostitutes. Consider the experiences of **Danielle**. Danielle was thirty-two years old
when interviewed and went as far as the tenth grade in school.
Danielle had used crack for only two years. She had never been married, but had what she described as a "common law" marriage with a
man who was in jail at the time. She and her boyfriend had been living
in a duplex apartment when the young woman who lived in the ad-
joining apartment allowed drug dealers to set up business there.

Enterprising Danielle saw a business opportunity and allowed the
people who purchased drugs next door to come into her apartment to
smoke for a fee in drugs or money. This eventually led to her boyfriend's arrest and incarceration. As a result she lost the apartment
and ended up homeless. It was then that she turned to selling sex.
Danielle became pregnant by exchange once. She was eight months
pregnant with this child at the time of the interview. The father of her
sex-for-crack baby is unknown. She has two other children. Her oldest is an eleven-year-old boy from a relationship she had after she left
high school. He was being cared for by Danielle's mother. A second
child, a one-year-old boy, is the jailed boyfriend's son. DFACS took
custody of him when she lost her apartment. Danielle describes her
first prostitution experience:

I needed some drugs and I didn't have no money. I had girlfriends that did
that [prostitution] and I knew how to do it. So I started going out on the street
and flag a car down. . . . The first time, this guy offered me twenty dollars for
sex. We had sex and he supposed to have gave me twenty dollars and he

gave me ten. I felt low, like a snake in the grass. And then, I wasn't used to doing that. I felt ashamed and nasty. It was my brother's so-called "friend."

Danielle was taken advantage of during her first prostitution experience. Being acquainted with the sex customer is no guarantee of fair treatment in the crack world. People who are involved in the selfish crack culture often maximize their gain at the expense of others.

Kathy was also the victim of a swindle during one of her early sex-for-crack encounters.

It was a hurting thing. I was about twenty-four . . . cause I learned a lot of shit when I started smoking. That incident was something. It was another young boy. I used to buy it from him so I figured it was the real deal. I got flexed [ripped off] after I bent over and gave him some and he got what he wanted. He gave me the stuff [crack], and after he left I put it on there [the fire] to smoke it. It wasn't even dope!!

The lines between prostitution for money and exchanging sex to support a crack habit were more blurred for women who had never engaged in prostitution before they became addicted to crack. These women had never earned a living through prostitution and had never traded sex in any other context. For them, obtaining money for sexual services was merely an intermediate step to obtaining crack. Some women suggested that as soon as the sex act was over the money was converted to crack so quickly that any time in between was irrelevant.

Furthermore, the men on the street, especially drug dealers, have become so accustomed to procuring sex for crack that they prefer to pay for sexual services with drugs. Paying for sex with money would give the women a sense of dignity and control. Thus, paying with crack denies the women these minimal sources of self-esteem.

Consider the experience of **Cybil.** Cybil was thirty-five years old at the time of the interview. She had several years of technical school and business-management training beyond high school, though her education did not translate into income-earning power. Cybil earned about $500 per month when she worked at a day care center. She had never been married. Cybil describes crack prostitution in the street:

I don't think there is a difference [between sex for crack and prostitution for money]. Because, when I prostituted, when I got the money, it was for the dope. There were times when I prostituted when they [men] had the dope. When I was on the street, the dope boys would be out there. When I prostituted with the dope boys, they never gave me money. They gave me dope.

They never give money; that was out of the question. They know that you are a "dope ho" and that if they do give you money, you will just give it back to them to buy some dope. . . . For me, I got to the point where I didn't care about anything else. I didn't care about going home or personal care, nothing. I didn't eat; I didn't sleep. When it got to that point, crack was my god. That's all I cared about. I didn't care what I looked liked, what I smelled like. I just wanted the dope.

When it got into that frame of mind, when I went out and seen the dope boys, they done already seen me buy dope before. Everybody knows who buys dope. If you go into this area, everybody knows that you are going to do dope. I was a known crack user. Eventually you are approached. Eventually somebody will say, "Yo, how much?" "You want to get high?" They can look at you and tell. . . . I can go out there right now and say, "That's one right there." If a woman is looking back or looking around, I know that she is either looking for a dope man or somebody to sell her body to. . . . It is such a habit to me. I still walk and look behind me today. . . . They know that if I'm out on the street I ain't got no dope, cause if I had some dope, I would be somewhere smoking it. . . . I was approached. "Yo, baby, you want to test this shit [dope] I got? You want to do something? You got some money?" I said, "All I got is me." Then, let's go behind this building, let's go in this bathroom, let's go in this car, truck, or in the bushes. Or I knew somebody. Money never came up. It was always for the dope. You look a certain way or carry yourself a certain way, and it's just oh, men. Everybody where I hung out at, except the people [who worked in the stores] did dope.

According to Cybil, women who use crack have a characteristic look or posture that men in the culture can easily recognize. Cybil accurately describes the state of crack prostitution on the streets today. The social scene is saturated with female crack users and it is a man's game. Any crack-using woman is approachable for sex without the slightest hint of etiquette or social graces. Men boldly get right to the point and ask "How much?" without an introduction or even "hello." To be sure, this practice has contributed to further sexual stereotyping of poor black females.

For poor black women, an extreme state of being sexually accessible to any man exists in the crack culture. Furthermore, gender-scripted social power of poor black females as heads of households and family leaders is eroded by the phenomenon as well.

One of the interesting paradoxes of first-time sex-for-crack experiences is that the women relished the attention they received for being the "new girl." Apparently, when a woman is a fresh face on the scene, many of the men who possess quantities of crack want to share their supply with her, romance her, or have sex with her. For some women, the first-time experience can be misleading. Toni gives a very eloquent description of her personal experience with this phenomenon:

I remember how when I got ready to turn my trick. I was the new kid on the block. I was sitting in the dope house getting high. I was so used to being spoiled, being a home kid, having everything. I was sitting in the dope house with jewelry on and outfits that my mother bought me. . . . I was so infatuated with all the guys that I thought were so cute and so "fly" in high school and junior high. Now here they is "dope boys" and I'm sitting here [in the crack house] and they are saying "Ah, man, we have a new girl!" I was getting all the attention. All the guys want to "kick it" with me. Give me some of their dope and some of their money. I thought that was the thing. I thought that I was gaining on the rest of the females because I had it all. Everybody was on me. It took a short period of time for me to realize that I was being used. I was being cheap.

Toni described the "honeymoon" phase for women who become crack prostitutes. The experience is the same for those who were once prostitutes for money. When a new girl enters the world of crack dealers and crack users she is usually considered potential fresh game or a new conquest. Many men are willing to share their drug supplies with her with the expectation that eventually a sexual barter deal will be secured. At the beginning of the honeymoon phase the women enjoy the attention and admiration of the men.

All too soon, however, the magic of that moment is over and sexual demands are made for subsequent money or crack. The sex may have initially occurred in the context of a mutual attraction. However, as with so many life situations, men and women approach this kind of sexual encounter with different expectations. The man, more often than not, is simply interested in sexual gratification. The woman may be interested in some kind of relationship with the man. Unfortunately, sex in conjunction with sharing crack with a man cements a woman's status as one willing to engage in sex for smoking crack. From that point on, a woman's grip on social power and respectability begins to erode.

Amy, who had prostitution experience before becoming a crack prostitute, makes this point clear:

I was fourteen when I started. When you are the new person on the block, them giving you stuff, that's how they hook you. It's like when you throw your line out to fish: you use bait. That's how that get you: with what they give you in the beginning. After that, you have to work for what you get.

The honeymoon phase ends very quickly. Eventually, women who exchange sex for crack are tolerated but viewed with disdain by men and even one another. When the charm wears off and the new girl becomes all too familiar, she must compete with the other women, either on the street or in crack houses, for a share of the crack bounty. The constant flow of new and younger women on the scene pushes the previous women out of the limelight. As the women who have "been around" plunge deeper into crack use and become more needy for the drug they are subjected to humiliation and ridicule. Sometimes the male crack holders refuse to sell to women who have become too familiar or too needy.

Kathy explains how these men treat women who have been "had":

Then they treat you like shit. Won't even sell you any. Tell you to get the fuck off. Treat you like no better than a cockroach.

Inner-city men who control crack harness power that they have rarely previously experienced. The rewards from possessing or selling crack in terms of income and social power give these men the dominance denied to them by the mainstream economic system. Being able to demand sex from a plethora of women who use crack, cast out women at a whim, and take charge of the social milieu is a heady experience for an unemployed black male. Toni reflects on the issue of power in the crack world:

They do it because it is a control issue, that power. I had a man tell me that "You know the feeling I get when every time I lay up with a woman for this dope and she gon' do everything I tell her to do because I got it, I got control. I got what she wants."

The more crack a man possesses or to which he has access, the more power he wields. Among men, high-level drug dealers are the most powerful and drug users are the least powerful. Bear in mind that high-level drug dealers generally do not live in the same neighborhoods as these women. Their visits are purely a matter of commerce. When a woman becomes involved with a prosperous drug dealer, quite often they are aware that these men have lives completely independent of their lives in the crack world. Several women expressed a kind of "wonderment" about the lives and relationships drug dealers had away from poor neighborhoods. Cybil describes, in vivid detail, the high-level drug dealers' operation methods:

They [the dope boys] are controlling people. They use these young black boys who stood out on every corner, on every store that sold beer. It was like a shift they used, until they sold out [of drugs], then they went back on their side of town where they lived a normal life over there. They are controlling and manipulative and they see women on the streets; we were their toys. Because whatever they said, we did. Even if they weren't getting ready to give us no dope, we did it. Because we knew that it might be possible that they may give us some dope. So if we knew that if he sold dope, if he said, "Yo, slim, come here" or "What you doing?" or "I got a boy that I want you to meet" or "Come and run to the store and get me something." We did it. Or rather, I did it, because I knew that if he didn't give me something [dope] right then, he might give me something [dope] later on. . . . They were show-offs. Flashy. Flashing money and jewelry, cars, their girlfriends—their young college girls that they would bring around us. It was degrading. And we would say [to the college girls] stuff like, "Y'all don't want to be like us. Don't do that shit [crack] he got." They would sit in their fine, pretty cars and watch us. And I don't think that they [college girls] knew what was going on out here. They knew that he [dope boy] was selling dope, but they didn't know what was going on with us out here. They couldn't possibly know.

This is when they [dope boys] would really torment us. [The dope boys said to the college girls] "That's a dope ho right there. I can get any one of them hos right now. I can have her suck my dick right now, in this car, with you sitting here, for five dollars." And he could! I wished he asked me to do it, because I would do it. If he ever asked, I would do it. I got to places where I would beg, "Please buy me." They [dope boys] brought their girlfriend around and showed out. They would leave them in the front seat of the car with the windows down. They [dope boys] would walk around with their pagers and cell phones and their jewelry and nice clothes, [with] pocketful of dope and a pocketful of money. . . . They're not going to let you know much more [about them] than that.

If you knew where a dope boy lived, if I knew where a dope boy lived, there was somebody in his family who used dope, either a brother or sister, or a girlfriend. Sometimes their girlfriends used dope, but they wouldn't let them hang out with us [street users]. Basically, you never knew where they lived. You knew where their dope houses were at. They never sat in that house. They would never let themselves be set up like that. They would never be in a confined area. They're going to be in a car, or they would be on the street somewhere. If they are [in a dope house], it's only for a brief moment. They ain't gonna be sitting up somewhere. They live across town.

Clearly, the men who possess large amounts of crack have unmeasurable social power in inner cities and the cash they generate provides a comfortable life somewhere, probably in the suburbs, far removed from the people they exploit. The young black boys they pay to act as street-level distributors garner power also, albeit to a much lesser degree. Dependent upon the situation, any man who has crack or the money to purchase crack has the ability to make demands of female crack users. The balance of power is tipped overwhelmingly toward the men in the crack culture. However, the women do exercise choices, such as partner selection and role negotiation (described later in the chpater), within a limited range to gain some semblance of control over their lives and to ensure their safety.

SEXUAL RISK TAKING

Women who exchange sex for crack risk contracting sexually transmitted diseases, becoming pregnant from anonymous partners, and contracting HIV by engaging in unprotected sex. Two issues were found to shape processes of sexual risk: early and traumatic sexual experiences and inadequate knowledge about sex and reproduction.

Early and Traumatic Sexual Experiences

Being born female into poor black communities is perilous. The sexualized image of black women and girls renders them vulnerable to sexual assault, molestation, and coerced early sexual experimentation. Sex is so taken for granted that early experiences are encouraged by peers. Most of the women felt that they were forced, pushed, or led into sexual relationships before they were ready. Some were molested as children or raped as adults. Some succumbed to pressure from an older boyfriend. The majority of women felt that they were not ready for sex at their first experience.

Most women in this study reported having sexual experiences well before the age reported by the majority of the population. Only two reported having sex for the first time at the age of eighteen or older. At the other end of the continuum, one woman reported having sex for the first time at age six. The others reported first sexual experiences between the ages of eleven and sixteen. A majority of the women entered sexual relationships immature and unprepared. April conveys how she first experienced sexual intercourse:

I was thirteen when I first had sex. It was with my boyfriend. It happened in the school yard. . . . We just wanted to find out what was going on. We didn't use protection because we didn't know to use protection. You know how children is, your mama didn't talk to you and you just didn't know no better. . . . I really didn't like it.

As mentioned before, both of April's parents were addicted to drugs when she was thirteen years old. As she indicated in statements presented previously, her parents were so preoccupied with crack that she began to raise herself in her early teens. She sought love and companionship with her middle-school boyfriend. Their curiosity about sex led to experimentation. Eventually, she became pregnant and left school. April felt that her mother did not arm her with enough information about sex and reproduction and she learned about sex only after having it.

Dena had her first sexual experience with a much older boy. She too felt that she was not ready for sex and knew nothing about it when her first experience occurred.

I was fifteen when I first had sex with my boyfriend. I cut school. I went over to a house in the projects, my girlfriend's mother's house. I was sore for two days. He used a condom. He was twenty-one years old. He was my girlfriend's brother. I liked him. I didn't like it [sex]. I didn't enjoy it. I didn't know what I was doing.

So many women in this analysis retorted, "I didn't know what I was doing" when they first had sex. **Valerie** expressed this as well:

I was fourteen when I first had sex. It was with a neighbor. We used to play together all the time. My brother used to have sex with his sister. He was about a year older than me. I didn't like it. It just didn't feel right. He was touching me and kissing me. He laid on top of me and just did it. I told him to stop, but to them no means yes. Yes to them means yes. I was the type of person who didn't know how to say no. I'm still like that. We didn't use anything. I didn't know nothing about it. I was young and I knew I wasn't supposed to be doing it. It was at my mother's house.

Valerie was twenty-six years old and had completed the tenth grade. She dropped out of high school due to peer pressure. Valerie indicated that her school friends influenced her to engage in behaviors such as skipping school. Her friends managed to graduate, but she did not. She became pregnant at age fourteen, but her mother pressured termination of the pregnancy. At age fifteen she became pregnant again and had the baby. Valerie had legal custody of this child, a daughter, at the time of the interview. However, her mother had been the actual care provider since the child was four years old. She had another child, a son, three years later. This child was legally adopted by an aunt and uncle at the urging of Valerie's mother.

Valerie's efforts to stop the neighbor's sexual advances were rebuffed and ignored. This scenario is rape. Cybil's first experience was nonconsensual as well. She was raped by a man who took her out on a date.

I was twenty-two when I first had sex. It was with some man. I hadn't known him that long. He raped me. It was date rape. We went out. I was really excited. It was our first date. He was much older than I. He said we were going to the movies. On the way, he said he forgot his money and had to go to the house. He said we could go in for a minute, have a drink, and listen to some music. It was fine. We go in and he bolted the door. I didn't think anything. I thought that he lived in a bad neighborhood, so he bolted the door. He proceeded to tell me that the music wasn't good enough in this room, so let's go in the back. I instantly thought, "Oh shit." I wasn't thinking "rape," but I was thinking that I was going to have to tell this man that I was not going to have sex with him. Let's just go to the movies. But it was a whole different story once I stepped in the door. Once I sat on the bed, it was over. He grabbed me and pinned my arms down and took my clothes off and raped me. I was crying and screaming. Someone came to the door, wondering what was going on. I got dressed and he took me back home.

I went in the house and shut the door. I sat on the bed and I cried. I didn't tell anybody. I didn't tell my sister. I was so embarrassed. I prided myself in my virginity because all my girlfriends were having sex. All of them were having babies. . . . I just wanted to forget it. And I did it successfully, until the next year, then I was raped again. I hadn't had sex with anybody inbetween.

Rape was a common experience for the women in the study. Fifteen out of the nineteen women had been raped at some time in their lives. Ten women had been raped more than once and one woman had been raped fifteen times. Four (Amy, Sylvia, Toni, and Dena) had been molested as children. **Sylvia,** age thirty-three when interviewed, had completed eighth grade. She reported having one sex-for-crack pregnancy: her four-month-old son, conceived in an exchange with a drug dealer. As a child, Sylvia was sexually abused by an older cousin. One woman in the study had her first sexual experience in the context of prostitution.

As mentioned before, Amy had her first consensual sex experience with a prostitution client.

I was molested at age six. I was thirteen when I had sex willingly. I had sex with a trick. He pointed me out [on the street] and we had sex. We used a condom. . . . I ran away from a foster home and ran into this guy. He introduced me to it, to being on the "ho stroll." I was about thirteen or fourteen. I was standing up on the stroll. A man pulled up. It was a bunch of us out there. But they always choose who they want. He pointed at me and I went over to the car. I remember having to be very careful in case he was the police. I had to let him proposition me. He propositioned me. He said he would give me forty dollars. We had a little house in the back, our pimp did, where we had two bodyguards in case the man got out of hand. He [the trick] had to pay ten dollars for the room for a certain amount of time. After he did all that, we went back there and we had sex and oral sex. He paid me straight off, because that's what you're supposed to do. We took care of business and he left. . . . I just did it. I didn't have any feeling or anything.

Too many of these women were not protected by their mothers or fathers in nurturing family situations during adolescence. They found themselves alone with older boys, unsupervised by adults, or on the streets. Many did not know about male-female relationships or how to express admiration without sexual involvement. Furthermore, with lack of parental supervision, they had few boundaries for boy-girl social interaction. Female gender vulnerability in volatile situations such as these superimposed upon them a sense of a lack of control over their own bodies. Most of the women in the study had very negative introductions to sex and were not informed about the mechanics of their bodies beforehand. Inadequate knowledge about sex and reproduction was a problematic area.

Inadequate Knowledge About Sex and Reproduction

Knowledge about sex and reproduction is divided into two parts: *early sexual knowledge,* which concerns how the women in the study discovered information about sex and reproduction in childhood; and *later sexual knowledge,* which assesses the extent of sexual knowledge at the time the women were interviewed.

Early Sexual Knowledge

In order to determine how the women first obtained knowledge about sex, menstruation, and reproduction, the following question was asked: "Who explained the facts of life about sex and reproduction to you?" Six women reported that their mothers explained this to them. Five women reported that girlfriends or others talked with them about sex. Eight women reported that no one explained the fundamental procreative processes to them.

The women were also asked: "How would you rate your knowledge about sex and reproduction at the time of your first sexual experience?" The possible answers were as follows: excellent, good, fair, poor, or no knowledge. The answers to this question varied with age of first sexual experience. The ten women reporting "no knowledge" at first sexual experience were very young at that time, ages six to fifteen. Only one woman, Cybil, said that her knowledge was excellent at the time of her first sexual experience. She was twenty-two when she lost her virginity. Unfortunately, she lost her virginity through a date rape.

Several women experienced having their periods before they were told anything about the changes that take place in a young woman's body, nor were they told anything about sex, relationships with boys, or pregnancy. Danielle explains how she learned about sex:

That was never explained to me. I just picked it up. I really learned most of it at school from friends. Once I started my period, everything just came to me.

When Kathy had her first menstrual cycle, she was terrified because no one had prepared her for it. She went to school and was embarrassed by her blood-stained clothing.

Nobody explained anything to me. My grandmother was old and the less I knew about it, the better. I didn't even know about periods. I thought I was pregnant. I wasn't even doing nothing [sex]. When I got my first period, I went to hiding in the closet. I took off the clothes and threw it under the bed. My grandmother said, "That's your period." She did tell me that. "You gon' have it every month. That means you ain't pregnant." That's as far as we got. I was eleven when I had my first period. I thought I was pregnant. I hadn't done nothing. I went in a panic. I went to school and messed up my clothes. I took my shirt and tied it behind me cause I didn't know nothing about no pads or nothing. I was so embarrassed. The teacher called my grandmother and told her that she should talk to me about my period. She eventually talked to me about it.

Sylvia's mother did not inform her about menstruation either. She received her education on the streets. Sylvia explains how she found out about sex:

No one told me anything. My mom, I don't think she wanted to be a mom. She never did sit me down to talk to me. I didn't even know what a period was. I love her to death, but . . . Eventually, she did come around and try to tell me, but I found out on the street. I've been having sex since I was fourteen. I was being abused by my cousin at about age seven or eight. . . . I don't remember my first sex experience. I guess you could say it was with my first baby daddy, my daughter. I was fifteen when I had her. I thought I was in love, but I wasn't. I found out that he was no good. . . . I was just doing something, I didn't know no better. I was very easy to be led.

These findings suggest that these women were not instructed to take control of the reproductive functions. They learned about sex and their own bodily functions by default. Though blame is a strong word, the women expressed disappointment that their mothers or other guardians had not talked to them openly about sex and relationships. In this part of their lives they learned by making costly mistakes that led to increased poverty and further restraints on life chances.

Later Sexual Knowledge: Assessing Sexual Risk Taking

Sexual-risk cognition was complex for these women for several reasons. Poor black females have a history of traumatic experiences associated with their sexuality and reproductive capability. This was evident in the lives of the women in the study. To place unprotected sex acts in the context of sexual risk taking and determine the prevalence of risk taking, the women were asked: "Did you use a condom with every trick?" All nineteen women answered no. Having firmly established this fact, three sets of questions were asked to evaluate the women's perception of risks they take when engaging in unprotected vaginal sex with tricks. The first question set involved sex and pregnancy, the second question set involved sex and sexually transmitted diseases, and the third involved the relationship between pregnancy and the fast-paced, crack-user lifestyle.

First, the women were asked: "When you are engaging in unprotected vaginal sex for crack, do you ever think about getting pregnant?" Only five women answered yes to this question. Furthermore,
the women were asked to explain the reasons for their answers.
Rarely does the thought of a possible pregnancy enter the mind of a
crack-using prostitute while a man is entering her body. The women
prefer to think about the crack they will receive or the crack that they
will purchase with the money they receive in return for the sex. Kathy
shares her thoughts on this subject:

I didn't use a condom. . . . I didn't carry them and half the time they [the men]
didn't have them either. I didn't think about that [getting pregnant]. That was
the last thing on my mind. When you are smoking you don't think about that
kind of stuff. All you want to do is [say], come on, I'm ready! I'm going to go
over here and this big one [rock] over here. "What you call them" got them
[rocks] down the street.

Again, the mental focus is on the drug. April echoes Kathy's remarks and goes further to describe her thwarted efforts to use condoms.

I didn't use condoms every time because I didn't have them. They cost and
the cost would take the money away from buying my crack. Then I start going to the health center and they would give them to me free and I would
wind up selling them to get crack then wound up without condoms. . . . Most
of the time that I would have vaginal sex without a rubber I would run in the
house and douche about four or five times. It got me back clean and got the
sperm out of me. Ugh. It's sick now to think about it. . . . I never thought about
getting pregnant.

April resurrects an old wives' tale about the effectiveness of douches
for preventing pregnancy.

The second component of sexual risk taking involved sexually
transmitted diseases. The nineteen women who participated in the
ethnographic component of the study experienced a variety of sexually transmitted diseases. Ten women reported one or more incidents
of syphilis. Fourteen women reported having gonorrhea one or more
times. Six women reported having outbreaks of genital warts, and
four reported having genital herpes. Eighteen out of nineteen women
reported one or more occurrence of trichomoniasis. Five women had
incidences of chlamydia.

The women were asked: "When you are engaging in unprotected vaginal sex for crack, do you ever think about getting diseases?" About half of the women (ten) said yes to this question. An explanation for the answer to this question was requested also. Living in an era when sexually transmitted disease can be resistant to conventional treatment or fatal, the concern for contracting sexually transmitted diseases was much more on some women's minds than pregnancy. Valerie, who was HIV positive, was naturally concerned about getting sexually transmitted diseases. She had already contracted gonorrhea, genital warts, chlamydia, trichomoniasis, and pelvic inflammatory disease.

I never thought about getting pregnant. When you are on crack, that is the last thing on your mind. Only thing you think about is if he going to give you the clap.

April thought about diseases also. She used her pregnancy prevention method—douches—to prevent diseases as well. As she indicates in the following statement, this method was not effective.

I didn't [use protection]. I used condoms sometimes. I had chlamydia, urinary infection, and trichomoniasis twice. . . . I thought about getting diseases all the time, every time. That's why I would run in the house and get me a douche bag and douche about three or four times.

The third question set provided the most interesting results. The women were asked: "Does the fast-paced, on-the-go lifestyle of a crack-using woman make her less likely to become pregnant?" Three women agreed with this assertion and the others disagreed. Explanations for their answers were also obtained. Toni, Sylvia, and Amy believed that the unstable lifestyle of a female crack user makes it harder for them to become pregnant. Toni describes the premise:

I do believe that women in the lifestyle get pregnant less. 'Cause most of the time when you are out there we have so many different men and what our bodies goes through. I feel like the reproductive system doesn't just work the same because you have sex so much. And you are on the go and are not resting and drinking enough fluids. You are always drinking beer and liquor. Rarely do you see people drinking water. The vitamins and nutrients that we need . . . we can't hold a baby. A lot of times we have these babies and they be dead. . . . But it makes it harder to fertilize babies with crack cocaine. When we do get pregnant, nine times out of ten the baby get knock right out.

Because we tricking so much and getting banged up so much by these men that the these babies don't stand a chance to develop; the egg don't stand a chance. I realize that . . . my body sure is flip-flopping. . . . A lot of times I thank God because . . . I know it has been several times, in there, that I have developed a child. But, moving so fast and beating my body down so much that it knocks it out.

Sylvia echoes the assertion that women who use crack are less likely to become pregnant.

If you have sexual intercourse and the man may ejaculate off in you, it doesn't do any good because the woman is moving so much that it [semen] is coming back down. You not really giving it time to sit for the egg to hatch . . . fertilize. So, constantly, I stayed on the go.

Amy believed that this factor was why she engaged in crack prostitution for many years and did not become pregnant, until the time of the interview.

It took me six years to get pregnant. I know I am pregnant now though. The baby I am carrying now, I don't know who the father is. There are a few that I had sex with around the time I got pregnant. That day, but which one it is I don't know who.

The other women vehemently disagreed with the premise that the lifestyle makes crack-using women less fertile. Kathy and Cybil share their ideas about the crack-user lifestyle and pregnancy. Kathy was particularly graphic in her comments:

I believe they do get pregnant [more often]. I think that they stand a better chance [of getting pregnant] 'cause they be running from dick to dick. Some of them just take the right one to just put it in there. Some of them [men] beat it up anyway. Some of them get in your stuff and don't want to come out; totally taking advantage of you.

Cybil took a pragmatic approach to the subject:

I think that they get pregnant more because they have sex all the time. They have sex every day in the month, practically. Even on their cycle they have sex. Not that you can have sex while you are on your period. In a normal relationship, you could miss that day [of ovulation] easily. When you are out there using, it's hard to miss that day, and if you're up under three months [pregnant] you can get free abortions all over Atlanta easily.

April shares information about female crack users and pregnancy from her perspective, and goes on to describe the results of their pregnancies:

Women [who use crack] get pregnant all the time. It's a lots of them walking around getting high and pregnant. Some of them get rid of them and some of them have them and give the babies to their kin people to take care of them.

The perception of sexual risk is juxtaposed against a background in which the facts of human sexuality were not openly discussed. When the women were children, most were not provided with enough information about sex and reproduction as they approached maturity. A majority were not informed or empowered to take charge of their bodies' functions or their sexuality. Some became sexually active without making a conscious decision to do so. This nonconfrontational approach to problem solving is a recurrent theme in the findings of this research. Rather than cope with the subject of sexuality, most of the women's guardians avoided talking about it until the issue was forced upon them.

Failure to confront the issue of potential pregnancy or sexually transmitted diseases is linked to the avoidance approach to sexuality learned in childhood. Perhaps guardians were trying to protect their daughters by shielding them from sex as long as they could, but in each case this strategy was not sufficient to circumvent traumatic sexual experience. The lack of knowledge may have instead had the opposite effect. When the women engage in unprotected vaginal sex for crack cocaine they prefer to rely on street myths or old wives' tales and even religious beliefs rather than become active in protecting themselves. The legacy of their early introduction to sex has left them with a sense of powerlessness to affect positive change in their behavior.

ROLE NEGOTIATION: PARTNER SELECTION, POWER, AND CONTROL

Despite the limitations on women due to their gender vulnerability in the crack social organization, many women actively constructed and negotiated roles for themselves. A few women in the study tried low-level drug dealing without much success. Those who attempted to sell drugs admitted that their profits literally went up in smoke. The women were much more successful at structurally organizing their prostitution activities in order to make the most money or crack and protect themselves against predatory men. They accomplished this with four mechanisms: (1) by developing conning skills, (2) by developing a tough street persona, (3) running a crack house, and/or (4) exercising some form of discretionary partner selection.

In descending order, partner selection was used by every woman in this analysis. All of the women had definite ideas about suitable partners and unsuitable partners. To be sure, the crack craving and level of relative desperation mediated the ability of the women to say yea or nay to a potential sex partner. Furthermore, most women admitted to having sex with at least a few men that under normal circumstances they would not. But, in many incidents, the women looked for a certain profile in their potential customers. Moreover, some women exchanged sex with only a number of regular "acquaintances" or established quasi-relationships with drug dealers.

Amy was one of those women who looked for a certain type of potential client. Her opinions coincide with views of the larger-society stereotypes concerning poor young black males.

One thing that I wouldn't do is turn a trick with a young black guy. Those are the ones that physically abuse and use you. Either they want to get on top of you and have rough sex to where its good to them but it hurts you or either they want to handle you any kind of way. Or give you soap [instead of dope]. This is why I focus on older men or men that are married, in high positions. Men that I knew could not afford to get caught and would not get mad at me taking their five hundred dollars, because of the publicity that it brings to your family or job.

Young black males who do not have the means to become high-level drug dealers are consciously avoided by many female crack users on the "ho stroll." Several women reported, as Amy suggests, that it is these men who practice packaging soap chips as crack rocks and attempt to obtain sexual services with these bogus substitutes. These men desire to obtain their share of the power along with the sex. Without the resources to purchase large quantities of crack legitimately, they employ this soap-chips charade to take advantage of the exploitative sex-for-crack barter system and momentarily harness the power endowed by possession of crack. These young men are often drug users themselves and are driven by the erratic crack craving as well. As the women have become aware of the men's fraudulent practices, young black males, disenfranchised within the crack social system, are shunned.

As Amy suggested, men outside the crack world who cruise inner-city neighborhoods looking for budget sex acts from desperate, crack-crazed women should think again. Many of these women are very intelligent, crafty, and are often after much more than the money agreed upon for the sex act. After spending several hours talking with Amy, I was convinced that if she obtained a good education she could have an excellent career as a politician or a judge. Her horrendous childhood prevented the accession of her obvious intelligence and people skills into something positive. Amy preferred to have several regular customers that she could meet at specified days and times. She describes her prostitution methods:

Well, you get dressed and you walk up on the "ho stroll." First, you make sure you get a meal, 'cause when you first come out you're hungry because of that strut you just came off of. You eat and you wash and you get pretty and make your way to the "ho stroll." . . . I would know what days and times to be where. I had regular dates. I had people that were regulars so I wouldn't have to jump in the car with just anybody. I would go to that spot. Say it was Tuesday, I would meet this certain guy on the corner of [X] and [Y] and I would be there waiting. At a certain time, he would drive up. I get in the car. I already know what he want and he already know what I want. We'd drive somewhere, like an abandoned piece of property, somewhere like that, and have sex, oral or either natural. He pay me and we leave. He drop me back off to the same spot and I go straight to the dope man. I purchase what I want. Then I go to the [dope] trap and stay in the [dope] trap or go to some-body's house and pay them to get high in their house.

When Danielle went out on the "ho stroll" she selected clientele according to the amount of cash they offered in tandem with the amount of work required. In the following quote she points out the very subjective analysis of any potential sex-for-crack transaction, and demonstrates the role crack cravings play in the decision-making process for many women.

It depends on who you get. They might say "How much do you charge for a blow job and sex?" You might tell them twenty-five dollars. Some might be willing to pay twenty-five, some might be willing to pay fifty. Then you might catch somebody who will give you ten dollars [for both oral and vaginal sex]. Then you might get someone who will want to give you five dollars for a blow job. But that is up to you to accept that. Or you could wait along until somebody else come up and maybe pay you two hundred fifty dollars for a blow job and this man gon' give you five dollars. It's up to you, how long you can wait, your patience. Till the right one come. If you want it [crack] real bad, you gon' take them five dollars. Or you will wait till another one come who will pay you more.

A few women exercised partner selection by juggling sexual activities with a small group of men that they knew fairly well or with casual acquaintances in their neighborhoods. What distinguishes these women from women with several boyfriends is the money or drugs changing hands. Consider the method of habit support used by **Chaka.** Chaka was thirty-nine years old, had completed the ninth grade in school, and reported earning less than $5,000 per year at a legitimate job. Chaka had become pregnant once by exchanging sex for crack, and the pregnancy resulted in a miscarriage. Chaka explains how she obtained drugs and money:

I had three friends. I had my children's daddy, the dude across the street, and my other baby daddy. I had got to the point where I go to my children daddy on Friday and get money from him. And then later that night, by the time I thought the dude across the street was home, I would go to the other and lay up with him and get money. And come Saturday I be done chilled out for a minute. Then I get the other baby daddy and go to the hotel with him. So one day I almost got caught with three different mens. I managed to play it off.

Rather than engaging in outright street prostitution, Chaka found ways to obtain cash from three different men in order to maintain her crack supply. A number of other women, including Valerie and Cybil, had relationships with drug dealers.

Valerie's father was a drug user, first of heroin and then crack, who spent most of his life in jail. She did not know if her parents were legally married. Her series of failed relationships with men produced her two older children. Valerie became pregnant by exchanging sex for crack on a regular basis with a drug dealer. This pregnancy resulted in her one-year-old daughter. Valerie had never worked longer than one month at legal jobs; at several fast food restaurants. Valerie was HIV positive though her children were free of the disease.

Her relationship with the drug dealer could be described as "loose." This dealer supervised a five-unit building in an apartment complex. One of the apartments was converted into a crack house. There was a minimum of ten girls/women working there. Valerie was not one of the regular girls. She showed up now and then to purchase crack. The regular girls recruited men from the neighborhood or the street to purchase crack or sex at the crack house. For five dollars more, the men could rent a room for sex with their choice of the women. Valerie regularly purchased crack from this particular crack house. Valerie describes the scene at her dealer friend's crack house.

The man starts it [propositioning for sex]. They [men] do their finger like that [come hither] and tell them to come here, pull them to the side, whisper in their ear. They may give my daughter's father five dollars. He was like the supervisor of one whole building. It had five apartment units. They would give him five dollars to use the room [for sex]. They would go in the room. There were at least ten girls in the house. The girls went out and made money and sit in the house and smoke in the house. . . . He [dealer] basically just sit there and smoke reefer. He would just sit there with all of us. People would come in to buy stuff. Some of the girls used to meet people outside that wanted to buy it; they bring them in. If they wanted to use a room to smoke, they paid him [dealer] five dollars to use the room.

Though Valerie was allowed to sleep at the house when she became homeless, she was not allowed to be one of the regular girls because she was not able to assume the street "get over" mentality completely enough. (The term *get over* is subject to a number of regional interpretations, but in general it represents achieving one's goals, especially at someone else's expense.) Apparently, the girls in the house regularly stole money from the men brought into the house. Valerie was terrified of doing this. She valued her life and did not desire to be beaten up or killed by some man for stealing his cash. The other girls ridiculed and cursed her. Valerie describes a typical day, explains the nature of her relationship with the girls in the house, and conveys the extent of her relationship with the drug dealer:

Well, I never got to sleep. From night to the next night to the next night I just be walking the street, smoking, trying to make money. . . . From the morning, I walk from one end of the block to the next end of the block. If somebody there already has dope, they call me to come smoke with them. Once I hit that, I come back out and walk again. I go to my third daughter father's [dealer] house and he has drugs. He'll tell me that I got to sleep with him before I get it. Just be sitting around all day, girls [in the crack house] cursing me out. Basically [the girls] not liking me because I didn't like to steal from nobody [in the crack house]. I wanted the drugs, but I was scared to steal it. I was scared that they would catch up to me and kill me. Then I really won't have no place to live. So they didn't like me and used to curse me out and put guns to my head. . . . Basically, if I go out there and make money, I'll specifically go back to my third daughter's father's house. I give him the money I made and he may give me two or three times as much as the money I gave him, just to assure that if I go out there and make some more money, I have to come back and buy from him and nobody else. I could always get it on credit, if he had it. . . . I used to get my drugs [for sex] from him and . . . [he] gave me a place to stay.

Valerie's description alludes to the very complicated relationships that have blossomed among crack users, dealers, and others in the culture. This dealer was someone Valerie purchased from regularly. When she was out of money she could exchange sex for the drugs she desired. The man had also fathered her youngest child. Although she was not considered his girlfriend, his generous allotment of crack to her indicates at least minimal favor. She did not think of him as a boyfriend or lover but rather as someone who sold her drugs and helped her when she was homeless.

As Valerie indicates, women must perform some kind of sex act to get the drugs, even if they have exclusively purchased drugs from that dealer in the past. This passage also supports the findings of other studies on street values (Stephens, 1991). The antisocial skill of stealing is a highly valued among the women in the crack house. Valerie's inability to perform in this capacity prevented her functioning as one of the regular crack house women. Values that result in social distancing by the mainstream of society are supported and encouraged by crack culture.

Cybil's relationship with a drug dealer was less tenuous, although it evolved into a violent relationship. She had never engaged in prostitution before she became involved with the dealer, whom she met in a serendipitous way. Cybil sustained controlled and orderly crack use for several years before the habit consumed her entire life. She managed to hold a job during the day, Monday through Friday, and smoked crack in the evenings and on weekends. A non–drug-using boyfriend provided her with extra money and a place to live. She used the funds from her job and from her boyfriend to purchase crack. Her boyfriend knew she was using it but did not intervene to keep her habit from escalating. In fact, Cybil felt he enabled her.

For Cybil, crack use eventually became an obsession. She loved what she described as crack's "intoxicating-like smell." Accordingly, continuing the meteoric high induced by the drug became her single passion. After she met her drug dealer friend her life began to spin out of control. Cybil conveys how her life changed when the man with access to dope entered her life.

I was going to my sister's house. When I got to her house, I noticed a lot a people standing around in the area. I was looking for a job. I had found a little job at Taco Bell or something. I pulled up to this house. I saw this guy and I knew he was a drug dealer. I could tell by the way he was dressed, the way he held his hands. I pulled up and said, "Anybody got any nicks or twenties or dimes?" He said, "We got some nicks," and I had like a hundred or hundred and twenty-five [dollars]. I parked the car, got out of the car, went in the house, and I didn't come out until the next week. This was like two blocks from my sister's house. I never went to pick him [boyfriend] up. I never called home, nothing. I seen that the dope was there; I had the money. I parked the car and went in the house and stayed. I stayed until it [the money] was gone. Once it was gone, I was asked to get the hell out of the house. I got in the car and went to the house [sister's] and went to sleep.

So the guy that sold me the drugs that night, he became my supplier. He immediately let me know that, "You can be my girl, as long as you take care of me sexually." At first, I didn't know how I was gonna do that and I don't know how I lasted so long, because I went to his house every night. We didn't have sex for about a good month or so. I found out later that was because he liked me so much personally; I didn't realize that. All I cared about was the dope. But eventually the sex did happen. And it was on a daily basis, sometimes more than once in a day. It got to he point that he liked me so much that he became possessive and he was jealous. It became violent. Even though it turned violent, I still did whatever he asked. I appeased him. Whatever it took, I did it. If it took oral sex, if it took staying in his room for eight days and not bathing, I did it. It got abusive. He would jump on me periodically, and slap me around two or three times a week. He kicked me, knocked me in the head, slapped me, knocked me down. He popped me in the mouth and talked to me any kind of way. He dogged me, but I allowed it because I wanted to do the dope. As long as I did it, I got what I wanted. . . .

He used dope, too. . . . He stole from his mother. He would get fifty dollars from his mother and buy a fifty dollar package and bag it up. He would sell what he could to get the fifty dollars back to buy another fifty dollar package, and that was over, that was usually sixty or seventy-five dollars over, to get that fifty dollars back. That's what he would smoke. It moved so fast; it was a continuous thing. After the abuse started, he busted me in the head, I mean busted me in the head. I bandaged it up and wore bangs, but I still stayed. . . . He lived at his mother's house. His mother sold drugs as well. Everybody in the house did drugs except the mom. It wasn't nothing but a crack house. His mother was about forty-seven years old. She is a big woman, she never left the house. She sold dope twenty-four/seven. That was her lifestyle. She never moved up [in the dope dealer hierarchy]. The more she made, the more her children stole from her. The house was beat up, with old run-down furniture. Nothing ever changed. The money her children didn't steal from her; that's what she made.

Cybil endured an abusive relationship in order to keep her crack supply going. But she always kept the relationship in perspective. This becomes plain in Cybil's subsequent statement. The preceding passage contains a classic example of low-level drug dealing in inner cities and demonstrates how crack lends itself to independent entrepreneurship. Anyone can purchase an amount of crack and try to sell it for twice the original price. This practice makes market-value control or assurance nearly impossible. The number of middlemen between the producer and the final consumer can be numerous. Furthermore, widespread poverty in inner cities encourages people of all ages to try their hand at the business.

Cybil's relationship with the dealer became more abusive as his attempts to control her failed and his drug use made him paranoid. After all, Cybil, who described herself as a "player," was still seeing her enabling boyfriend occasionally and continued to obtain money from him as well. Her independence was difficult for the drug dealer to handle. When his masculine authority was threatened, he used a ploy extremely prevalent among males in the crack culture: he cut off her crack supply. Deprived of crack for any length of time was unfathomable for Cybil. She turned to prostitution quickly, to keep her perpetual high. Cybil explains:

After the abuse started, he got to the point where he would cut me off [of the drugs]. And I would sneak out the back door. One day when I was sneaking out the back door, the tenant that lived downstairs caught me. I said, "Oh, shit!" That's when I turned my first trick. That was the first time I sold my body to somebody besides him [dealer boyfriend]. I sold my body for ten dollars. I had no problem with it. I was so happy to get the ten dollars.

So from there, if he cut me off, I went to the streets. I went out the back door. No matter how I looked, no matter how I smelled, no matter how many times I had sex with this man [dealer boyfriend] without a condom I went out the back door. The only time I used a condom was if the man asked. If he didn't bring it up, I didn't bring it up.

. . . This [the first-time prostitution] was three years ago. I was thirty-one [years old]. We [Cybil and boyfriend dealer] were on a binge for about seven days. After you have been smoking crack for so long you start to see things.

After you have been awake for so long you start to see things differently. Hallucinations begin. He had a thing where he thought I was fucking all the time. Whenever he walked in the room, I had to freeze. Because to him, if I was moving, I was fucking. He came into the door one night. I was sitting on the couch and listening to music. He said, "I see you're fucking, so I'm cutting you off right now. You're not getting no more dope for eight hours." When he left out, I went out the back door. I didn't want to go for eight hours with no dope. I crept down the stairs. The guy that lived downstairs seen me. He went through the regular routine. He said "Psssst, I been watching you. It [sex] must be good, 'cause he don't let you come out [of the house]. I got ten dollars." He knew that I had been up there for days. [I thought] To hell with it! I went in the room, took my clothes off, got in the bed, and had sex. Thank God I didn't have to have any oral sex. I got the ten dollars, sneaked around the corner, and bought me some dope. . . . I hate oral sex, but I had to do it a lot.

This woman refused to allow the drug dealer's restrictions to stop her from enjoying her passion for crack. It was simply a matter of walking out of the door to find another man willing to give her money for her crack habit. In inner-city neighborhoods, women who use crack have become so linked to sexual activity that men are comfortable approaching them with cash in hand expecting to be accommodated. Cybil's experience shows that the men are not often disappointed.

Easy sexual accessibility has been a crushing blow to poor black women's status in their communities. Male-female relationships not based on mutual crack use or some form of exploitation are nearly impossible for crack users who exchange sex for crack to maintain. Lack of trust, jealousy, and suspicion are common among both men and women who have become intimate with each other in the crack-use context. It is well known that people who use crack will generally do anything for the drug. Thus, few people trust their partners to be faithful. Crack also produces a paranoia that enhances mistrust. Cybil's drug dealer partner experienced extreme paranoia and mistrust concerning her. Her partner's mental state, coupled with Cybil's behavior, changed the nature of their relationship. Cybil explains:

Some guys come over to the house. We were having a "smoke out." That means you smoke till you say ah huh. . . . He [drug dealer boyfriend] kept mirrors all around the house so he could watch me. He was so paranoid. When he was out in the kitchen, the guys were coming on to me. After they left, I knew something was fin' to change. He was mad. He said, "From now on, you gon' have to fuck for yours [dope]. If you want yours [dope], I want it [sex] every day. That way I know you won't be fucking no one else." Like that would make a difference. I could have sex with him ten times a day and still have sex with somebody else. . . . He said that you are my woman now. Before I was just his fuck partner and we shared dope. That's when it changed. He changed the rules. He said now you are fucking for your dope. Now you will work for this. I had to do whatever he said. Now I was his woman; I had to do anything he said. Wash his clothes, clean up, whatever, I had to do it. Be quiet, go to the store, whatever, I had to do it. That's when it really started changing. Once he said that, it changed.

I would come over and he asked, "How much?" I would tell him, "I want one nick to smoke now, two to smoke before we have sex, and two afterwards." Each nick is five dollars' worth [a total of], twenty-five. That's what would happen. I smoked a nick first. We would have oral sex, which was me doing him. I didn't want him to do me. We had sex any way he wanted. Thank God he never wanted anal sex. But if he had, I would have done it. While we were having sex, he gave me two nicks. While he was performing on me, I was fixing my shit [dope] up. It was very difficult to do. I would have to say stop for a minute or slow down so I could take it [dope] out of the bag. Then afterwards he would give me another two. He would be in a good mood after that and everything would be fine. Then later in the day, if he wanted to have sex again, I would just have to do it.

Flirting with some men at a party and likely her indiscretion as well contributed to a dramatic change in their relationship. Cybil's relationship with her dealer changed to strictly exchanging sex for crack to much more. He made certain demands of her and she complied, just to maintain access to the drug. In contrast, the dealer considered her "his woman." In Cybil's mind, she entered into the relationship to be near a steady crack supply, and in this way she was exchanging sex for crack. The dealer, however, did not make that connection until later in their relationship. For the dealer, elevating her to "his woman" meant that she would function in the capacity of a common-law wife. At the same time it meant that the crack she received from him was payment for sexual acts. Even more confusing is the man's insistence upon asking Cybil, "How much?" as a man would ask a prostitute. This was probably a ploy to control a very independent woman. Perhaps in asking her the question the dealer's intent was to humiliate her or put her in her place. Cybil's experience in the dealer's house demonstrates the complex nature of sex for crack.

The lines between a quasi-relationship and prostitution are indistinguishable in many cases. In the crack world, prostitutes and women appear to be synonymous labels to some men, and men who seek to control women with crack are not always as successful as they would like to be.

Cybil became pregnant three times by the drug dealer. She aborted all three of the pregnancies. A fourth pregnancy was carried to term. Cybil is not sure whether the dope dealer is the father of her sixteen-month-old son or if it is her enabling boyfriend, though she admitted that she had sex with the dope dealer much more than with her other sex partner. She had had sex with the dope dealer two to three times per day during the period she became pregnant. Furthermore, she reported using birth control methods when she had sex with her boyfriend.

The drug dealers Valerie and Cybil stumbled upon were low-level drug dealers. These dealers had access to large amounts of crack, but not enough to allow them to have sufficient income to advance upward in the distribution network. Their customers were their families, neighbors, acquaintances, and friends. Acting in interest of themselves, community-based drug dealers sell a destructive commodity that exacerbates the disintegration of their own neighborhoods. Both women became involved with the dealers to get closer to crack supplies. The dealers were very different in their approaches to the women. Valerie's dealer was not a crack user. He managed to exercise more control over his life and over his relationship with Valerie by keeping her at a distance. Cybil's dealer used crack. This may have contributed to the abuse that she underwent. It also may be related to Cybil's triumph in resisting his efforts to control her. Gaining control over one's life in the crack world can be difficult. Some women maintain a sense of balance and normalcy in their lives by defining and limiting the geographical space for crack use or prostitution and by using that space to generate income for themselves. Both Danielle and Toni operated crack houses.

Before engaging in prostitution, Danielle supported her drug habit by allowing other people to come into her apartment to smoke. At first she allowed crack users access to her home without asking for payment. When she discovered that money could be made, she charged a fee in drugs or money to enter. Danielle shares how she started and describes the organization of her crack house and its rules:

I ran a crack house. I found out how to run a crack house through my brother. I rented him a room and he smoked in it. So he practically told me how to run the house. I used to let them come in and smoke for free. I was smoking too.

Until he told me that when they come through the door, tell them that they had to give a house hit or a sack [of crack]. So when they came through the door, according to how much they had, like they had one dime [ten dollars' worth], they had to give me a house hit. If they had more than ten dollars' worth, they had to give me a dime, a whole sack; a ten-dollar sack. So everybody who came through the door had to give me a house hit, a sack, or money. They had to bring something. Somebody I knew real good, I might let them come in [for less]. They might say, "I don't have but this [amount of money]. And I'll say come on in. . . . I might let some people come in for a quart of beer or some cigarettes. They might say, "I brought you this, but I ain't got nothing but this dime or this nickel bag [of crack], but I brought you this beer." . . .

I had a room that they could have sex in. It was five dollars for thirty minutes and ten dollars for an hour. If they wanted to pay me in crack, instead of giving me five dollars for thirty minutes, they would give me a dime bag. If they wanted an hour, they would give me two dimes for an hour.

Most people thought I was mean 'cause I would put you out in a minute. If you got too loud, I'd put you out . . . then, if you come in just to smoke and you don't want to rent the room, there was a time limit. If you got a ten-dollar bag of dope, I might let you sit there no longer than an hour. Then, I'm gonna put you out! 'Cause you ain't gon' just be sitting around my house, sitting there waiting for other people to come in so you can beg. Those were my rules. According to how much dope you got, how long you can sit. If you ain't got but five dollars [of crack], I might let you sit there thirty minutes. It don't take that long to smoke that. Take about five or ten minutes, probably not that long. So I'll put you out. I had a time limit for how long you could sit there. . . . No peeping out the windows. No standing at the door. No in and out, running in and out the door, no traffic. It was kept quiet. . . . They couldn't use my little boy's room. My mother took him away. . . . It was good because I didn't have to trick at the time. It was coming to me. That's why I used to tell my old man that "I don't see how those girls go out there and do that." Not long after that I did have to go out there. When he went to jail, that's what put me out there [on the streets].

If a woman has an apartment in the inner city or in public housing, where drugs are plentiful, running a crack "smoke" house is a way to take advantage of the flow of people cruising the neighborhood looking for drugs. This simplest form of crack house does not require much, only a shelter and a willingness to let strangers in. Danielle did not sell drugs or engage in prostitution at that time. She allowed people who purchased drugs from the dealers next door to smoke in her place, and rented rooms to other women who turned tricks. These kinds of arrangements have proliferated all over inner-city neighborhoods. So many people are drawn into some component of the crack-selling and underground-hospitality industry that, as indicated previously, small children are exposed to drugs and prostitution at very young ages. Authors such as Elijah Anderson (1990) have likened these establishments to the speakeasies the prohibition era in America. On the contrary, speakeasies were adult business establishments, whereas all too often crack houses are set up in homes where children are present.

Danielle's crack house was organized and administered similar to many others. In most crack houses, customers are restricted to a specific area and are given a time limit. Moreover, when the drugs or money are gone, the customer must leave the premises. These rules are nearly universal in crack houses.

Danielle became homeless after her common-law spouse was incarcerated. This drove her to do something she vowed she would never do: prostitution on the streets. For Danielle, running a crack house was a way to avoid prostitution. In contrast, Toni's crack house was a way to enhance and embellish her business as a sex worker. Toni describes the sex and drugs business she established in a hotel:

Most of the crack houses that I've been in have been in hotels. They would have the setting where there was a room and you have the tables for the smoking and music. The TV, but nobody watches TV. Women would have candles lit to romance the men and make them feel comfortable. For me, I would section my room off. I would use the bed for the tricks and this part over here for the smoking. You have traffic, so much, after you get the popularity of your room. Men get used to coming in and not worrying about getting ripped off, that's how I kept mine [room].

I had a room in a hotel. I lived in a hotel. This hotel was basically a crack hotel. The manager, the owner knew this. That's how she got paid. Even the security officer got paid like this. It went by floors. The first floor was for businessmen, women, and for families. The second floor was for businessmen who wanted dates and didn't want people to know about it or who wanted to use [drugs] privately and didn't want to be bothered with all the traffic. The third floor was for drug dealers, prostitution, and anything illegal. If you were found out being wide open, participating in this [illegal acts] on the first or second floor, the manager would move you to the third floor. They wouldn't put you out. They would just move you.

This is like the underworld. Since I been here in Atlanta, this is where I stayed. It got to the point where I was selling so much drugs and sex that I was able to afford three rooms at one time. I kept one room for prostitution and dates, one room for drug dealing, and one room for my own comfort, for my privacy, my activities. That's how I got my first case for selling drugs. I got busted for possession of two ounces of cocaine. . . .

When I first started learning how to do it [cook cocaine powder into crack] and I realized I could profit rather than helping these drug dealers, I would help other drug dealers on the side because they said, "Darn, Toni really has this business going." I would always dress appropriately. Not like a business-woman in a bank; but everything had to be perfect. I would not smoke crack unless my makeup was done, or unless there was alcohol around because you wanted to get these guys comfortable. Relaxed and okay. . . .

[Where do the men come from?] There was a truck lot outside the hotel. And not just that, this industrial boulevard, [X] Industrial Boulevard is well known for this activity. The cops know and they get paid from the prostitutes. This is how it goes on [X] Industrial. It's so known for it. The business is so good. The companies and stuff. It's all businessmen. To attract Indian men, Arab men, and black men with money. My thing was always white men. I would always stick with white men or foreigners. There's money to be on the "ho stroll" and get regular customers. Because of the way I dressed, all the time money was so easy. I recall being on [X] Industrial and I had my schedule. I would go to work just like everybody else. I would sleep all day and about when the sun went down, I would go out about six o'clock in the evening. And I think I would clock out at about ten. From six o'clock to ten, on good days—Thursday, Fri-day, and Saturday—when I counted up my money, I would have eight hundred to a thousand [dollars]. In one day, I would have about two hundred fifty. . . .

I would always have somebody working with me, because you see these fe-males and other drug users and know that this is the thing. You got dope dealers that like your style and the way you do things. They would always come to you and drop some of their dope off and let you solicit it to, some of their drugs, to men who are attracted to your room. The ladies that would come around, I had no problem with having client workers. They were using and dealing for a profit. They saw the money that was being spent. It was amazing. You had more drug dealers hanging around your room like they were using drugs. Everybody wanted to get a piece of the pie.

After eleven o'clock at night, on the weekdays, I would pay the security offi-cer twenty dollars per customer. They came off the truck lot. You had just as many white men as black men. The majority of the dates, the guys that use [crack] were white men. Just the setting, being with a black woman that they could trust, they loved that. Just to come in and be romanced, and all this. It was amazing. Guys would come and sit and spend their paychecks or in-come tax checks for days and never leave. They would just stay there. Guys would come in with the intention to go to work. They would call in [sick] and just for days [stay]. Especially when the income tax [refunds] come out, at this hotel, I profited so much. I was blessed. I made so much money, but where is it?

Toni operated an efficient drugs sales and prostitution enterprise. She was highly organized and attentive to detail. Having learned about crack at the beginning of the epidemic, she also knew how to cook powder cocaine into the formidable rock. This skill enhanced her ability to produce income. Her business grew as she attracted men from varying backgrounds and income levels. According to Toni, for a time the business was highly successful. As her own crack habit intensified, however, she began to smoke away her profits.

This is a common pattern among crack-using women. A number of the women in the study reflect on times when they were able to manage their lives with getting high. Eventually, using the drug became so important that the other parts of their lives were neglected. Toni's experience is a good example of this phenomenon. The hotel in which Toni's enterprise was situated was known for drugs and prostitution. As indicated, even the security officers at the hotel were a part of the underground network. The hotel was organized around illegal activities, with many people openly coming and going at unusual hours. Since this kind of activity is normal for the area, Toni must have become careless as a result of her drug use. She was eventually arrested for possession of a relatively small quantity of cocaine. This was out of character for her. Toni was very intelligent, perceptive, and extremely well organized in the way she conducted her life. Drug use took its toll, and she lost her lucrative brothel and her role as proprietor.

Using crack heavily makes it impossible to function well for extended periods of time. Danielle and Toni created roles for themselves in the crack underworld that maximized the amount of cash they could make, maintained a stable living environment, and kept the crack supply coming, at least for a season. Crack house operations such as these require resources and specific social skills. Not every woman was able to accomplish having her own crack house, but they learned other ways to survive in the crack world, for instance, most of the women in the study developed defensive skills to protect themselves from predatory men.

Danielle and April developed tough street personas in their dealings with men. The principle behind the tough street persona is simple: if women are as treacherous and tough as their male associates, then potential harm or the potential for being taken advantage of is reduced. As discussed earlier, some men attempt to obtain sex from women without paying. Crack-using women also are raped and beaten up routinely.

Danielle explains how she and other women avoided physical harm and ensured that men lived up to their end of any bargains.

You just have to get bad with them. "Give me my goddam purse." Fight them back. You practically have to be dog just like they're doing. You treat them like a dog the same way they're doing you. When they see you ain't no joke, nothing to play with, you can kind of get what you supposed to get. 'Cause some of them try to do you like that and all the time they're scared. This woman have power. But they see you ain't the one to be messed with. They're gonna give up what they're supposed to give up. But some of them, some men just gonna dog you out. A lady can't handle a man unless she got a gun on the man. That's the only way.

Danielle admits that men have the physical advantage over women, and this factor limits the application of the tough street persona, but many women try it. Sometimes it is successful at thwarting a rip-off artist and other times it is not. Another variation on the tough street act is the crazy street act. When the situation with a man becomes difficult or the gets out of hand, some women feign insanity. They pretend to be high on crack and in a state of temporary lunacy. Some women take this ploy a step further and use it to rip off the men. After first smoking crack with a man and finishing the high, some women want to avoid following through on the sex act that is expected. As the prospect of having sex becomes more repugnant, the women put on an act that spoils the mood. April, for example, garnered a nickname for her tough and bizarre street style.

I don't give them a chance to [humiliate me]. Most of the time I trick them. I tell them that I am going to give them some sex if they let me go on and smoke this [crack] or give me the money. When they do that, I get high and act like I'm all geeked up. Then, they say shit, she ain't gon' do nothing. Then they leave. . . . Men used to call me "do dirty" because I will grab me a knife and fight and say, "Give me my money!" Men have done me like that, but they wind up giving me my money. They call me "crazy." I do not play about my money. If I done did what you ask me to do, you gon' pay me my money. Or I'll die first. And I want that crack too. If I want that hit bad enough, they gon' pay me. . . . I have ran off with the money many times.

The tough street persona is closely related to the practice of conning. The men in the crack culture are not the only perpetrators of rip-off schemes. Many of the women in the study resented performing sex with the men so much that they incorporated conning techniques into their daily prostitution activities. Conning involved promising to have sex in exchange for crack or money and then reneging on the agreement. Another form of conning involved taking money from someone desiring to purchase crack and absconding with the cash. Sylvia was especially good at conning clients. She had practiced prostitution as a teenager and came to loathe the oldest profession, so she developed a smooth conning technique. When that was not effective, she quickly adopted the tough street persona.

Some men and women enjoy being ripped off. . . . I have ripped them off. I would lie and promise sex and wouldn't do it. I would stay right in my area so if anything go down, somebody is there. Knowing I wasn't going to do what I said I was going to do anyway. Then I would get smart and say, "Nigger, you a sissy. I wasn't gonna fuck with you no way!" Then he would say, "I will kill you." Some people enjoy that. They enjoy them taking your money. I have had people to come back, knowing I was the same girl who took their money last week. But they come back and try it again. Then I take their money again. Some people get tired of you taking their money and telling them that you will be right back, knowing that you ain't coming back.

Sylvia justified her actions by believing that people enjoyed being robbed and deceived. She could be right. Both sexes in the crack world practice this kind of swindling. These games are primarily played between inner-city black men and women and can be an extended venue in which the battle between the sexes is fought on a daily basis. The men rip off the women and the women retaliate by ripping off the men. The women expect the men to pay for sex; the men expect the women to provide sexual services. In many cases, both men and women attempt to get something without living up to their end of the bargain. All violate the "rules." In the crack world, rules are always for someone else to follow. Most people justify their own con games while deriding others for engaging in the same behavior. Each gender imposes expectations on the other that they could not live up to themselves. When a woman is focused on the business aspects of sex-for-crack prostitution, she may seek to avoid the aforementioned sexually charged acts of fraud.

Toni, Amy, and a few others targeted white men, married men, or affluent black men in order to avoid falling prey to sexual swindles. Toni elaborates on this issue:

When they see a lot of women going out doing the dope would get abused and used like this, it got to a point where women were robbing the men and men were found tied up because, speaking for myself, I had gotten tired of it. I got to the point that I even would get my money up front, and a nigger would beat me down and take my money back. I remember when I started really doing my thing, I thought, if I can't get one, I'll get the next one. I got where I would get with white men or foreign men or older black men. I would make sure I had a man with status or that was married. I wanted to know something about you so I could blackmail you. And I was good at it. My skills at blackmailing were so good, not knowing that I was taking a risk of getting killed.

For most women, even obtaining the money or crack first was no guarantee that they would avoid a swindle. Sylvia's previous description of conning methods points out why men may be reluctant to give the money or drugs to a woman before the sex occurs. It is a no-win situation. Trust is completely lacking. Predatory behavior among the women increased as they became victims more often. Concomitantly, as women victimize men, men feel vindicated in victimizing women. Thus, in the crack world there is no peace. Being victimized and victimizing others is a way of life. Toni preferred clients with status, but, like Amy, found that blackmailing these men was a way to make even more money than by prostitution. Though she moved to another class of men, she took her crack-world mind-set and values with her.

Regardless of which strategies are used by crack prostitutes to improve their lot, sooner or later the crack addiction consumes so much of their time that they are unable to maintain the most basic functions and life stability. Partner selection and other methods of protection are abandoned. The difficulties imposed on the women by their limited lives and by crack compulsion have a direct impact on their responses to sex-for-crack conceived pregnancies.

Chapter 7

Sex-for-Crack Pregnancies

THE WOMEN AND THEIR PREGNANCIES

Sex-for-crack pregnancies occur in circumstances unimaginable for bringing a child into the world. The mothers are indigent and drug dependent and involved in a dangerous, unpredictable, underworld subculture. The pregnancies begin in an atmosphere of trickery, treachery, mistrust, exploitation, and degradation, and within a complex matrix of potential fathers. The fathers of sex-for-crack children could be drug dealers, acquaintances, or strangers, to name a few. In this study, a significant number of pregnancies were brought to term and resulted in offspring to mothers who had too few resources to sustain themselves let alone an infant. Out of forty-one sex-for-crack–induced pregnancies among twenty-three women, only seven were electively aborted. Probing deeper, the ethnographic interviews suggest that three issues shaped responses to sex-for-crack pregnancies: (1) severity of crack use, (2) religious beliefs, and (3) the social organization within inner-city poor black communities.

ISSUES INFLUENCING PREGNANCY RESPONSES

Severity of Crack Use

Severity of crack use appears to be a primary force in determining the response to a pregnancy. Preceding pregnancy, severity of crack consumption also influences the chances of a sex-for-crack pregnancy occurring. As indicated earlier, daily crack use was commonplace for most women. One of the major difficulties for these women was focusing on anything other than the immediate need for the drug. In the absence of crack or any other addiction, the harsh realities of poverty will often keep individuals focused on day-to-day survival. Crack use has exacerbated the daily survival mentality by shifting the focus to moment-by-moment survival. Crack use is associated with compulsive, repetitive behavior that impairs the ability to think beyond achieving the next high. In this way, crack use truncates thought processes and allows only immediate phenomena.

The repetitive cycle of geeking and freaking—using crack (geeking) followed by performing sexual acts (freaking)—followed by more crack use eventually consumes all or nearly all of the users' time. April describes the process of geeking and freaking:

It's [crack] easy to get. I really didn't go to sleep. I slept every now and then. I used to stay out, twenty-four/seven, getting money, getting drugs. I never really stopped. I just do it constantly. I get up in the morning—or really never sleep—I just wash up and get ready to go out again, find a man, have some sex, and get me some more crack, and do it over and over again. I smoke the crack at a friend's house, the same house I go to every day. Might as well say eat and sleep at, when I do eat and sleep. It's a crack house. I just go out over and over again. It's like a circle. Every day: Monday, Tuesday, Wednesday, Thursday, Friday, Saturday, Sunday.

Crack-using women are constantly on the go for days at a time, either using crack, finding someone who will give them crack or the money to buy crack, or performing sexual acts until their bodies are exhausted. This cycle makes it difficult for women to manage their bodies, their lives, and the lives of their children. The drive to get high again and again motivates women to take unacceptable risks. One such risk is performing sex without contraceptives or protection.

The women report that while engaging in unprotected vaginal sex for crack cocaine, the thought of the consequences of such behavior—pregnancy or sexually transmitted diseases—is crowded out by the anticipation of experiencing the immediate reward. Kathy describes her experience:

You don't be thinking about that I might get pregnant or that he might have the clap. You only think about "come on, so I can go and get my rock!"

The crack high is a powerful motivator for users to do what they believe they must to get the drug. The fast-rising HIV epidemic among black women in general may be linked to the increases in transmission among poor black female crack users who engage in drug-related prostitution. As indicated earlier, Valerie was HIV positive at the time of the interview. She performed unprotected sexual acts, vaginal and oral, with tricks. Valerie explains:

I didn't use a condom with every trick. Sometimes if you don't have one, the trick is not going to wait for you to go buy one. If they are one of those persons who believe in using condoms, they stop to the store to buy one they self. But most of the time, they didn't. They just wanted to do what they got to do and be gone.

Valerie placed her clients at risk for HIV infection every time she performed sex without a condom. Her HIV status was never a consideration in changing her behavior. Crack use creates such an urgency that self-protection strategies are rarely invoked. Another respondent, Danielle, explains why condoms are not used on a consistent basis.

I did not use a condom with every trick. One, because you're ready to smoke crack, and two, because you don't have one and he [the trick] don't have one, or the guy don't want to use one. And you willing to let him go ahead and do it because you want a hit; you want a smoke real bad. So you say, "Okay, come on then, you ain't got none [condom], come on. Let's get this over with so I can go and get me something to smoke." I really don't want to touch him, but go on and do it and get it over with and get off of me. . . . Practically, I have to think about something else. You do what you have to do. There's no feeling in it. For me, there was no feeling in it, none whatsoever. It just, you just want to get through with it. But you got to do what you gotta to do to get that crack 'cause you want it just that bad. I think about getting crack [while having sex]. That's what you have to think 'cause that's why you're out there doing it. You think about that next hit and that makes you go on and do it and get through it, the quicker you get that hit.

Men who pay for sexual services with crack prostitutes are playing Russian roulette with a fully loaded gun. Some of the women are HIV positive and most of them are exposed to many sexually transmitted diseases. Safe sex is not practiced consistently among this group of women.

Focusing on the euphoria that the crack will bring motivates the women to complete the sexual act as quickly as possible in order to continue drug use. The future consequences of such acts are unacknowledged in favor of concentration on the immediate reward: another crack cocaine rock. Similar to Danielle, a number of other women in the study expressed disgust at the prospect of having sex with some of their clients. They relented and completed the acts but kept their minds on the anticipated crack high. The sexual activities are barely tolerated by many women. Crack helps them escape from the thought of the unsavory characters who demand sex for small amounts of money or crack.

Toni echoes the sentiments of many others:

When you do use [crack], you just want that hit then and there and you ain't got time to get no condom. You just want to get this [sex] over with so you can get your next hit. You say [to the man], "Hurry up and get this over with and get up off me so I can get my next hit."

In the beginning of the crack epidemic, oral sex was the act most frequently requested by men on the streets. It didn't take long for more demands to be placed on women and often for much less cash or crack cocaine. Cybil explains the crack prostitution situation as it existed in the late 1990s:

Actually, practically every man would say, "You've got to get it up first." By that they meant that you would have to suck it first. That was just the norm. They wanted both [vaginal and oral sex]. The main line was, "You've got to get it up first." That means you got to suck it first. They wanted vaginal sex every time.

Vaginal sex became the more common request from crack prostitution clients. Ten of the women in the ethnography component of the study ($n = 19$) indicated that the men on the street demand vaginal sex half of the time or more. When asked to estimate how often they performed unprotected vaginal sex with tricks in an average week, four women answered once or twice per week, six women answered three times per week, five women answered four or five times per week, three women answered daily, and one woman answered more than once daily. For Toni, the request for vaginal or oral sex varied by the type of prostitution customer. She makes a distinction between drug dealers and tricks on the street:

Eighty percent of the men like vaginal sex and you got twenty percent that want oral. There is a difference between tricks on the street and drug dealers. A drug dealer wants oral sex because most of them are dating their girlfriends. They think that it [oral sex] is safe, so they think. They think they can't catch anything. Now, most tricks on the street who pick you up want vaginal sex because of the money that they spend. They spend more money, they want the whole nine yards. They [dealers] can give you a hit and that's it or a sack for oral sex. They used to have twenties and fifties. Now they got dimes and nickel rocks. They give you a nickel rock and you think this is the whole world. Especially at late night hours when things done went down and you want a hit of your own stuff. A lot of times you want your own and don't want to use someone else's bag. You just do something [sex] for it and they will give you a sack for oral sex.

The drug dealers basically do not give a flip. To get money from a drug dealer, he has to be an older man. You catch a few young guys that want to be with this woman or this trick and might give you money if none of their friends are around. But, they won't give you money in front of them; the drugs is the power.

Under these conditions: the age of the women, high-volume vaginal sex, and no protection, pregnancies are inevitable. Severity of crack use interferes with responses to the physical condition of pregnancy also.

After becoming pregnant by exchange, one of the most common responses to the situation is to ignore the pregnancy and increase crack use. Moreover, some women continue to focus on moment-by-moment survival and fail to make any decisions about the future of the pregnancy. The pregnancy simply continues, without prenatal care, proper nutrition, rest, or any other health care practice usually prescribed for pregnant women. When Cybil, Dena, Danielle, and Linda became pregnant by exchanging sex for crack, they all ignored the changes in their bodies and plunged deeper into crack use.

As indicated earlier, Cybil had four sex-for-crack pregnancies. She aborted the first three. The fourth time she became pregnant she was unable to tear herself away from using crack. Cybil reports the story of what happened after she became pregnant the fourth time:

I had the baby because I was too lazy. I did not want to stop [using crack]. I was so small that I convinced myself that I was not pregnant. My baby hardly moved, if ever. I never ate. The only time I ate was after days of doing dope. I would be so tired. I can't tell you how many times I fell asleep eating, literally, and wake up with food in my mouth; in my bed; in my hands. You know I could have died. I could have choked to death.

I wore my regular clothes. It was cold so I could camouflage it really well. I was in denial about the pregnancy. Then one month, I had a [menstrual] cycle. I said, "Oooh, I'm really not pregnant!" But I really was. Then the next month I didn't have a cycle. Then the next month I had another cycle. I said, "Oooh, I'm not pregnant." The baby didn't move. I could feel a lump. My stomach would growl like I was really hungry. My stomach would do that and I thought that was the baby, but that wasn't the baby. Then, after about five months, that's when the baby started moving because I got heavier into the use of crack. Real heavy. I had an abundance of it. When I wasn't using, he [the baby] used to kick my ass. Once I used, he was all right. Then he'd get in one position and just hold it. When he was an infant he would do that. Just get in one position and hold it. I got pictures of him doing it. They told me that was the withdrawal.

I carried him seven months; I used seven months. I had one day of prenatal care on Friday and I had him that [next] Monday. He weighed three pounds eleven ounces. They kept him [in the hospital] for two weeks. He did well, considering how small he was. He was breathing ninety-eight percent on his own. They were truly amazed. They asked me how long I smoked dope and I told them every day. The only time I didn't smoke dope was when I was asleep.

Remarkably, Cybil's son lived in spite of in-utero drug exposure and premature birth. This child was sixteen months old when Cybil was interviewed. She indicated that social services in the state (DFACS) removed the baby from her custody earlier in the year and that was the last time she had seen him. Her sister had custody of her seven-year-old daughter. Her daughter was not conceived in a sex-for-crack deal. Cybil articulated very clearly the denial present for a notable number of women who became pregnant exchanging sex for crack.

Dena also continued her crack use after she became pregnant. She had two sex-for-crack pregnancies. The identity of the children's fathers remains a mystery.

I had my daughter. I didn't know I was pregnant. I was just out there. I just didn't give a damn. She is three. I don't know who the father is. . . . I didn't take time to do nothing about it. . . . I was out there in the street. It was the crack. I was not responsible. . . . I am pregnant now [by exchange]. I really didn't handle the situation, I was too far gone. I am seven-and-a-half months pregnant. I don't know who the father is. I waited too late [to have an abortion].

Dena's mother had custody of all three of her children, including the three-year-old daughter. Danielle explains what occurred with her sex-for-crack pregnancy:

It wasn't planned for me to keep the baby. . . . I was supposed to be having an abortion, but by me smoking crack every day I just couldn't seem to get myself to the doctor. I kept saying, "I'm going tomorrow to have an abortion." I kept putting it off until I just kept getting bigger and bigger. Then I was too far gone. . . . I don't know who the father is.

Danielle did not desire to be pregnant under these circumstances and wanted to terminate the pregnancy, but her addiction held her captive in the repetitive cycle of crack-related activity. This made it difficult to prevent the birth of an unplanned child of unknown paternity. She delivered her child, though she used crack during a significant portion of her pregnancy. She managed to obtain custody of her sex-for-crack–conceived baby by remaining clean in the last trimester of her pregnancy. Her two other children were in the custody of others: one with a relative and the other in state-ordered foster care. Another respondent, **Linda,** had similar experiences.

Linda was thirty-seven years old at the time of the interview. She completed the eleventh grade in school and dropped out of school after she became pregnant. She reported earning $1,000 a month from prostitution. She had never been married, and, similar to the other women in this analysis, Linda had a series of unsuccessful relationships with men, including a drug dealer. She had two sex-for-crack pregnancies. The first pregnancy was fathered by the drug dealer and resulted in a stillbirth. The second pregnancy was fathered by a married man who gave her money for sex and resulted in the birth of her now one-month-old daughter. Linda shares the events of her first sex-for-crack pregnancy:

I didn't get no kind of prenatal care. I was going with this guy who sold dope and smoked dope. He didn't care. If he cared, he would have stopped me. I was eight months pregnant, I think, because I didn't know when I got pregnant. That Friday I wasn't feeling good. I was smoking. I kept vomiting. I kept smoking, not caring about the outcome of it. That Saturday my baby was still moving. Still getting high and stuff. That Sunday afternoon I didn't feel my baby moving. I said it probably ain't nothing. That Sunday night I went into labor. I called the ambulance and they took me to Grady. They did the ultrasound and the baby didn't have no heartbeat. The baby was stillborn. I was in love with this man who didn't care nothing about me. He was a [drug] dealer.

Linda used crack for five months while carrying her second sex-for-crack child and she managed to get several months of prenatal care before delivering her daughter.

Denial of sex-for-crack pregnancies and continued or increased crack use is a familiar pattern. Kathy and April reported responding to their sex-for-crack pregnancies this way also. Another response to becoming pregnant by sex-for-crack exchange linked to severe crack consumption involves the physiology of a woman's body and the pregnancy itself. Some women believe that becoming pregnant can provide a relief from having monthly menstrual periods and give more time for exchanging sex for crack. When individuals engage in sex as often as do these women, having a menstrual cycle can be a challenge. A number of women reported that they simply continued to have unprotected vaginal sex during their periods and invented creative explanations to appease the men. Most acknowledged that their lifestyle made it difficult to manage the female reproductive bodily functions. Cessation of menstruation due to pregnancy may be considered a means to provide more time to exchange sex for crack. April shares her view on this subject:

I got sick and didn't know I was pregnant until I was about three months. I was too busy smoking. I didn't care about the sick symptoms. I didn't pay it no attention. I was still trying to get out money to get crack. I didn't pay none of it [her menstrual cycle] any attention. That made it better on me. Not having a period, I could go out and get more money to get crack.

April also suggests that discomfort associated with morning sickness did not deter the pursuit of the crack high. During the early months of pregnancy, ignoring the symptoms and continuing the crack-user lifestyle is easier. Once a pregnancy is obvious, denial is no longer possible. Even after a pregnancy is very obvious, some women continue to focus on using crack rather than coping with their physical conditions. Kathy was one of those women. She was eight months pregnant with her second sex-for-crack–conceived child and she continued to smoke heavily. This child, a daughter, was born in a crack house as Kathy continued to use crack and ignored her obvious labor pains.

I delivered my baby in a crack house. I still have a problem dealing with that. Her head was coming out and I was steady trying to buy me another rock. And now she suffer with asthma real bad and I know it is my fault. That will be with me until the day I die, because I did that. Crack cocaine messes up and destroys and takes away a lot of stuff. The hardest part about it is that you want to keep getting high, thinking that's going to ease the pain, and it helps a little bit. But once it's down, and speaking for myself, that's why I keep constantly wanting to get high, because the problems still be there—a lot of things that I didn't want to deal with that was happening in my life because of that. So I steadily kept smoking to ease the pain.

This extreme case demonstrates the power of crack and shows how it is used to temporarily shut out reality. After it was clear to Kathy that she was in labor, she had a choice of going to the hospital or going to a crack house. She chose the latter. The impending birth of her child was not enough to stop the desire to be high again. Kathy became pregnant by sex-for-crack exchange three times and carried each pregnancy to term. They were ages seven, six, and two at the time of the interview. She also has three older children. All of her children, except the youngest, were in the custody of her relatives. At the time of the interview she had custody of her two-year-old.

The act of delivering a child in a crack house demonstrates the power of crack to strip women of ordinary commonsense practices. April shares a similar experience concerning delivery of her sex-for-crack baby and her inability to stop crack use:

I used crack all the while I was pregnant. I was in labor, my water broke, and I was still trying to smoke. That is so sick. I feel so guilty.

These examples make clear the severe nature of crack addiction for poor black women and the dangerous consequences of crack addiction on reproductive potential and on children.

The three women who chose to have abortions indicated that intense crack use was closely connected to their decision to take action. As mentioned earlier, Cybil aborted three sex-for-crack pregnancies sired by her dealer friend. She indicated that her desire to remain high motivated her to make the effort to have abortions.

I had abortions because I didn't want the babies. I wanted to continue to smoke dope. I didn't want the responsibility. Matter of fact, it was so hard for me to stop smoking to go and have an abortion. . . . The dope boy was the father of all three pregnancies.

The controlling influence of crack is demonstrated by Cybil's experience, but she managed to break free of the cycle on three occasions and aborted the sex-for-crack pregnancies. Her desire to continue smoking was powerful motivation for the abortions, although she acknowledges that this same desire also made it hard to find time to go to the abortion clinic. For Cybil, and for most of the other women, severity of crack use played a critical role in the occurrence of sex-for-crack pregnancies and served as a major influence over the pregnancies' outcomes as well.

Religious Beliefs

Sex-for-crack pregnancy outcomes are also influenced by religious beliefs. Deeply rooted spirituality deterred some women from obtaining abortions. All of the women who participated in the ethnographic interviews reported a belief in God. Most believe that God provided protection for them in spite of their behavior. When faced with a drug-trade conception, divine inspiration sometimes motivates women to carry the baby to term. April shares her experience:

I never thought about getting pregnant. I didn't want no baby from those men. I just didn't care. . . . I was too busy trying to smoke, getting money to get crack, or get crack to smoke. Yes, it bothered me, but when I did get pregnant, it was what the Lord wanted. If the Lord didn't want me to get pregnant, I wouldn't have gotten pregnant.

The women make a strong connection between God and the conception of a child. They were administered a series of eight true-or-false answer statements to gain a sense of their knowledge about basic human reproduction and their feelings about it. One item from the list was: "Babies are conceived only by God." Fifteen women answered "true" to this question. To help themselves accept a sex-for-crack pregnancy, several women attached spiritual significance to the child.

Recall that Linda had two sex-for-crack pregnancies. The first was stillborn. Linda believes that God gave her a second chance with her second sex-for-crack pregnancy. She relates the loneliness she felt and the hope that the baby would fill a void in her empty life:

It was a mistake. I didn't plan her. She is one month old. God gave me a second chance. I have always wanted a little girl. It was like God was saying you need something or somebody in your life to change you. I believe God put my baby there to change my life. . . . Her father is a married man. He came to see me in the hospital. . . . He was a trick to me. Every time we would have sex he would give me money. I have custody of my daughter. I wanted the baby. I was in love with the man and wanted a baby by him. I was alone; my [oldest] son is grown. I know that is one of the reasons I do crack. I was lonely. Depression sets in.

The women in the study lived extremely unfulfilling lives before crack use. Crack is often used to numb the feelings of loneliness and inadequacy felt by being poverty stricken in a wealthy country. Rather than helping, the crack consumption makes the marginalization worse. Women cling to religious beliefs in order to maintain some hope for the future.

Religious beliefs and church activities have long been associated with black life in America. Traditionally, black women have occupied central roles in church organizations and ceremonies. One of the consequences of the emigration of middle- and working-class blacks from inner-city neighborhoods is the change in church accessibility for poor blacks remaining in the city. Churches that formerly served black neighborhoods during segregation have either moved to the suburbs or have gradually become *commuter churches.* Commuter churches are churches located in inner cities for which the majority of their congregations live in the suburbs and commute to attend services on Sundays. The commuter-church phenomenon is a critical development in current inner-city social conditions all over the United States. These churches generally have significant histories in black neighborhoods, and many middle- and working-class blacks maintain ties to their families and ancestral spiritual roots by attending the churches of their childhood. The congregations of these churches, for the most part, are not the impoverished city dwellers. There are exceptions to this trend, for example, the Nation of Islam, which concentrates outreach efforts to the poor, but the pattern of traditional black church gentrification is clear.

Poor black female crack users are frequently estranged from the churches of their childhood. Nevertheless, church affiliation and denomination membership remain an important part of their self-definitions. Furthermore, women invoke the religion-based definitions of self when faced with a sex-for-crack pregnancy. Kathy vividly emphasizes this definition:

I was f— everything and not using no condoms. I had the baby because I am Baptist and I don't believe in killing. . . . When I found out [I was pregnant], I said "God." But I constantly kept getting high. I don't want no abortion. I don't know who the daddy is. I didn't want to kill it because I don't believe in abortion.

Religious beliefs and spirituality remain an important part of poor black women's lives, but their neighborhoods provide little institutional support for the formal expression of these sentiments. In the past, neighborhoods and communities were built around church membership. Churches served as help centers in which the pastor and congregation actively involved themselves in the needs and concerns of the surrounding community. Now, many inner-city churches draw their congregations from a variety of geographical locations. Most of these church members live in other communities, pay taxes in those communities, and have an interest in bettering neighborhoods far removed from their religious institutions.

Commuting to church on Sunday is a once-per-week activity. Thus, many inner-city black churches are closed Monday through Saturday. The poor people who live in these neighborhoods, especially crack users, are deprived of a venerated social institution that once figured prominently in sustaining poor blacks. Another hallmark of poor black communities plays a role in the outcomes of sex-for-crack pregnancies: Social-organization structures were found to influence choices made by women who became pregnant.

Social Organization within Poor Black Communities

The third influence on the outcome of sex-for-crack pregnancies is the social organization of poor black communities. The prevalence of single-parent, female-headed households was evident among the majority of the respondents' families. The women rarely knew much about their fathers. Even if their parents were legally married, divorce, separation, and early death fractured family stability. Even more influential, a pattern of mothers' disengagement from family life was discovered.

The Legacy of Mothers' and Fathers' Relationships

The project participants' mothers and fathers had difficulties achieving and maintaining traditional marriages. Their mothers' sexual relationships with a series of partners, some of which produced other children, created severe strain on home lives. Most of the interviewees had siblings outside of their family groups by their mothers, fathers, or both. Many of the women in the study describe situations in which their mothers' and fathers' changing relationships with the opposite sex pushed their children into the care of others. It became apparent that most of these women spent significant amounts of time alone and unsupervised during childhood. Some even reported raising themselves.

Consider the families of Sylvia, Toni, Cybil, and Dena. Their experiences show a variety of family patterns that have one thing in common: difficult home lives as children that involved the transfer of child-rearing responsibilities to someone other than their parents.

Sylvia's background was one of extreme poverty. Her mother worked as a domestic and lived in public housing. Sylvia lived with her aunt until she was seven years old, until her mother "just snatched" her from the custody of her aunt. Sylvia describes her early family life:

My mother and dad were not married. She was married to someone else. But she had me. My dad was never in my life. I knew who he was. He's dead now. This man my mother was going with, that's who I call my father. . . . My aunt raised me. . . . There are six of us. I have two sisters and three brothers in all by my mother. I have a brother and sister by my dad. I don't know nothing about them.

Sylvia's life on the street began early, at age fourteen. Young and impressionable, and feeling that her mother did not want to be a mother, she followed the practices of the other young girls in her neighborhood and engaged in prostitution for money and in shoplifting. At age fifteen Sylvia started using marijuana daily and drinking alcohol. Lack of parental supervision and overreliance on peer-group relationships for social support left Sylvia with few guidelines for her behavior. She became involved with a group of people who robbed and burglarized routinely. Sylvia reported an affinity for breaking into cars. Her introduction into substance abuse and street crimes in childhood made the transition into the crack world easy. By the time she tried crack for the first time, at age twenty-two, she was a seasoned veteran at illegal activities. She found little difficulty supporting her crack habit with prostitution and stealing.

Toni's family life was difficult and confusing as well. Her mother was married to her sister's father when she became pregnant with Toni. Toni did not get along well with her mother. Their relationship remained strained even after Toni reached adulthood.

My mother and father were not legally married. My mother was married to my sister's father. He went off to the service. He became shell-shocked. My mother got with my father. I have one sister by my mother. I have three sisters and one brother by my father. . . . I lived with my aunt. Me and my mother never got along.

Her difficulties at home stemmed from changing family composition and her father's job as a drug dealer. She didn't know much about her father when she was very young, but came to know him later. His involvement with drug sales and burglary were a powerful influence on her subsequent involvement with illegal activities, and later on the organized way that she approached prostitution. Toni became involved in shoplifting in expensive clothing stores as a young teenager. She attributes her involvement with shoplifting to her father. She reported seeing how "simple" it was for her father to obtain money and material goods by stealing, so she decided to try it for herself. Crack entered the picture when she was eighteen years old.

Recall that Dena was the product of an unmarried teenage mother.

My mother got pregnant when she was fifteen with me. My father was her boyfriend. She said she thought he looked good. . . . My parents were not married. . . . I have two sisters by my mother and a brother. One sister and brother by my dad. My grandmother raised me.

Dena lived with her grandmother until her grandmother died. She later went back to live with her mother. However, when Dena reached eighteen years of age, her mother withdrew any responsibility to Dena. Her mother helped her find an apartment and paid the rent for two months, after which she told Dena she was on her own. Shortly thereafter Dena became homeless.

Cybil's early life was extremely unstable as well. Her parents divorced, after which her mother moved from place to place, sometimes taking her children with her and sometimes leaving them behind. Cybil describes her family life:

My mom has moved around since I was about ten [years old], without us. She would leave and go to this state and that, here and there. I lived with my big sister; she raised me. My parents were married, but they divorced in 1962. I have three sisters and one brother by my mother and dad. I have one brother by my dad.

Cybil felt frustrated with her mother's inability to keep a job in one place to provide some stability for her children. She indicated that she thought her mother was "paranoid about life."

Fathers' and Mothers' Role Ambiguity

The preceding descriptions underscore the findings of many studies conducted in the 1960s and 1970s on poor black families. These studies were discussed in Chapter 2. Parents' serial relationships, which produced children, may result in complex families and male parental role ambiguity. As mentioned earlier, the fathers of poor black children are often not consistently involved in their lives. This phenomenon is typical for the women in the present study. Few knew much about their fathers. However, the data show an increased tendency toward their mothers' role ambiguity in family life. The women in the study were frequently raised by grandmothers, aunts, and others. The heavy reliance on the extended family for the upbringing of children also supports the earlier studies' findings on poor black families. The generational downshift in responsibility later played a central role in the women's responses to their own children. The women did not express much anxiety about not knowing their fathers, but when their mothers were not able to care for them, they experienced deep emotional scars. Most women expressed subtle, if not open, disappointment with their upbringing and family situations. They felt their mothers did not provide adequate training and did not spend enough time with them.

When a poor black mother is unable to take responsibility for her offspring, and no grandmother is available, poor black children are fortunate if a relative can raise them. The pool of stable extended family members to care for children has declined as the prevalence of substance abuse has increased.

As discussed earlier, social and economic pressures on poor black men have contributed to their decline in family-life participation. Before the introduction of crack, the tension between men and women increased as marriage rates decreased. Sexual conquest without commitment became a primary goal for many young men. Conversely, achieving commitment from men through sexual favors became the hope of young women. These conflicting goals have the socially devastating consequence of children born without a supportive family network, to young, ill-prepared parents. Married couples with children are now the exception rather than the rule among this demographic group. Women generally bear the sole responsibility for supporting and caring for children. Fatherhood for many men is a status in name only. The gender roles associated with fatherhood, for example, provider, disciplinarian, and masculine role model, are intermittent, transitory, and ambiguous. Thus, women have low expectations for the men in their lives. Dena sheds light on the meaning of fatherhood in a brief comment:

I don't know what it means to be a good father.

Both Valerie and April agreed. It was difficult for these women to conceptualize an image of a good father since they did not have positive male role models in their lives. April's father caused his entire family to be crack addicted. She was especially bitter toward him for that reason.

The sex-for-crack barter system and the resulting pregnancies have taken the ambiguity of male gender roles to an extreme low. Possessing quantities of crack enhanced the social power of jobless men and boys in the inner city. Men who possess crack have the power to demand sex from any crack-using woman without responsibility, commitment, or respect. Most women report having sex with men with whom they would ordinarily not associate. For men, achieving sexual conquests is just a matter of obtaining crack cocaine. Inner-city men have used crack to exploit and humiliate female crack users, and thus have further strained the tense relationships between men and women. As word spread that inner-city neighborhoods were sources of budget prostitution ($2 or less), the pool of males desiring sex for either crack or money widened to include suburban black men, white men, and many others. Sources of male genetic material for sex-for-crack pregnancies are broad, but sources for women of male economic and social support are narrow or nonexistent. Having a child conceived by sex-for-crack exchange emphasizes the lack of concern for biological paternity. Women prefer to concentrate on the child and not the conception. Kathy expresses concerns about her children having a legal father, though the actual paternity of each child is unknown.

I have two of them [sex-for-crack conceived children]. I got pregnant and I don't know who their fathers is. I thank God that my husband and I were still married so they're still in his name and he claims them. But up to this day, I don't know who they [the fathers] was because there were so many of them.

Although Kathy was separated from her husband, she was still legally married to him and could place his name on the birth certificate of these children and legitimize their births. Women sometimes feel trapped between two conflicting sets of cultural norms: the norms of mainstream society and those of the inner-city community. The norms of the larger society stress the importance of marriage for the well-being of children. The realities of inner-city poverty make marriage for most black women difficult to achieve and maintain. However, as Kathy's story indicates, women may harbor ideals about marriage and desire legitimacy for their children but are resigned to the limitations of their circumstances.

Social and economic changes in inner cities that have occurred over the past thirty years have established the single-parent, female-headed household as the predominant family-composition pattern and exacerbated male disengagement from procreative responsibility among poor blacks. Having a child by an absent father has become the norm rather than the exception. This phenomenon occurs independently from drug use. Thus, poor black women who become pregnant by sex-for-crack exchange live within a sociocultural system in which the role of a child's biological father is not of primary importance. The importance of children is stressed, not the circumstances of their conception. For these women, having a child by an unknown father appears to be no more shameful than the mainstream practice of having a child by artificial insemination. In addition to not having a clear image of a father role model, most women did not have a clear image of a mother role model either. They were asked, "What does it mean to be a good mother?" Most women delivered short, abstract, and unfocused answers. Dena's remark was typical of most other women:

Being there for my kids.

April provided one of the most comprehensive and focused answers to the meaning of motherhood:

It means a lot to be a good mother. That's what I am trying to be now. It means taking care of my kids, cooking, washing, cleaning, and doing things with them. Going to school, doing projects with them, hugging them, letting them know I love them.

For most women, their perceptions of motherhood were based on negative experiences with their own mothers. Estrangement from their mothers, their mothers' substance abuse, their mothers' changing relationships with men, neglect in childhood, or unstable home lives made the roles associated with motherhood unclear. With limited societal roles to occupy, motherhood is important for the women's self-definition, yet few of them have a decisive pattern of behavior to follow. In fact, strained relationships with their mothers were cited as the cause of crack use for some. Amy felt that her crack use started in reaction to rejection by her biological mother. Recall that her mother gave Amy and her brother up for adoption when they were babies. When Amy finally met her mother, it was a disappointment.

I was about nineteen. At that time my life was in turmoil. I had met my biological mother at age eighteen. She abandoned my brother and I from birth. We meet her and once again, she abandoned us. I had nobody. The guy I was living with left me for another girl. He left me with an apartment and a lot of bills. I had this one best friend. I knew she was using it [crack] but she would always come to my house when she was living with her mother. And she came there and she went to the bathroom. She was in there a long time. I was laying in my bed just crying and crying. I went to the bathroom to see if she was all right. She had been in there for so long. She hugged me and said don't worry and that it was going to be all right. Then she said "try this." So when I tried it and I immediately got the feeling that, I got numb. All my pain was gone. The hurt was gone. All of a sudden I didn't care that my mother had left me or that my boyfriend had left me. I was just all right. The misery was just gone. I felt good. I immediately made a decision to let that [crack] be my medication to get rid of my pain. And because of that I kept doing it. I got addicted. I had to have it. I would go to any lengths to get it.

An unexpected finding in this analysis is the trend toward mothers' disengagement from the family in the previous generation. As mentioned earlier, half of the women in the ethnography sample were raised by someone other than their mothers or fathers. Furthermore, the move to the extended family did not stabilize the women's lives. These findings contradict earlier studies about the strength of the extended family.

CHILD LOSS

A majority of women (fifteen) had lost custody to either family members or through state intervention. Some had lost children before involvement with crack. Recall that eight women dropped out of school due to pregnancy. In some of these cases, the respondents' mothers took custody of these children. Furthermore, some women had abortions, miscarriages, and stillbirths that were not related to sex-for-crack pregnancies. The women were asked: "Did losing a child to abortion, miscarriage, stillbirth, or legal or family intervention influence you to become pregnant again?" Based on the women's answers child loss did not appear to motivate the women to become pregnant again. The pregnancies seemed to occur because the women did not feel empowered to take control over reproduction. Valerie conveys her thoughts on this subject:

I don't think that losing a child influenced me to become pregnant again. My mother took custody of my nine-year-old at age four. My aunt and uncle took custody of my six-year-old at birth.

When I really started smoking crack real bad and was spending my check and food stamps on it, and the rent money, I didn't have food in the house. I knew what the people on the street was going through. Having somewhere to live and not pay my rent, just feeling like if I can't pay my rent, I knew they would put me out. So I just left. . . . I was living with my mother when I was pregnant with my son. My mother said that I had to figure out what I was going to do, "'Cause you still living with me you can't live with me with two kids." So she called my uncle and aunt and asked if they would adopt my son. I felt like I was forced into it. . . . It hurt a lot to lose my children, but I was grateful because if she would have stayed with me, DFACS would have had her. At least she was with a family member and I can always see her.

April had lost all of her children due to the incident of child abuse described earlier. She became pregnant less than a year after her children were taken. However, she felt that the loss of her children was not related to her additional pregnancy. April explains:

I lost all my children to DFACS. This happened a year ago. The fifteen-, thirteen-, eight-, and seven-year-olds. Four boys. This happened in May of 1997 after the thing happened with my sister. They just came in and took all of our kids. . . . I became pregnant again, in October of 1997. I don't think that losing the children influenced me to become pregnant again. I just got pregnant. I just didn't use protection. [About losing the children] I didn't like it because—I was using drugs true enough—but I was taking care of my kids. My kids went to school every day. They was clean and they ate good, every day. I just was doing one thing wrong: I was using drugs. Sometimes I left, but I wasn't gone long. My sisters were there. My twin sister. I didn't leave them with my little sister [Carrie] that did all of this stuff. I left them with my twin sister. Or I left them with my daughter. She is big enough girl. She would watch them until I came back. She don't use drugs; she don't smoke. She don't go to school. She is pregnant. . . . I didn't like it [losing the children]. Did you see me on the news? I was cussing and going on. I wanted to fight.

April had also had an abortion at age seventeen.

I had an abortion when I was seventeen years old. The father of the baby was the father of my first two kids. I wanted to have an abortion. The Lord is against abortion. I didn't have no bad feelings 'bout it. It's just a child didn't know. I wish I hadn't.

Only one woman thought child loss influenced additional pregnancies. She lost her children to death. Toni had two children die in infancy. She grieved the loss of these children and believed that her additional pregnancies were conceived to fill the void that their loss created.

The consequences of crack addiction for poor black women are far reaching and severe for them, for poor black families, and for communities. The compulsive nature of crack addiction makes condom use difficult and renders women vulnerable to unwanted, unplanned pregnancies by men with whom they have perfunctory relationships, have no relationships, or whom they do not know. The crack-addiction cycle keeps the women focused on moment-by-moment survival to the exclusion of taking control of their bodies, reproductive potential, and their children before, during, and after birth.

In this sample of women, exchanging sex for crack indeed results in pregnancies. Abortion of a sex-for-crack pregnancy was a rarely chosen option. A common initial response to the pregnancy was denial. It is clear that the women did not desire to become pregnant by a prostitution client, but they did little to prevent it from occurring. When it did happen, they continued to use crack, sometimes up to the very point of delivery, placing themselves and the baby in jeopardy. The way these women embrace the crack high—as though they have nothing to lose—highlights the interacting dynamics of race, class, and gender marginalization among this group as well as the powerful appeal of crack for uplifting the spirits, if only for a few moments. The women have become accustomed to a limited range of choices, constrained by poverty, female sex, and black ethnicity.

Motherhood is often the women's only source of life satisfaction. In black communities, especially poor ones, motherhood is endowed with power, status, and strength. Becoming a crack "ho" greatly diminishes this culturally based social power. The large numbers of women who exchange sex for crack in inner cities, and in particular the significant numbers of those with children, has damaged the status of motherhood in these communities. Having children by prostitution customers may have damaged motherhood as well. One literature source, Inciardi and colleagues' (1993) *Women and Crack Cocaine* suggests that in some cases, sex-for-crack–conceived children are referred to as "trick babies" on the street (Sharpe, 2001). The interviewed women strongly identify with motherhood, but a number of paradoxes are made apparent by this research.

Some of the women interviewed expressed guilt about using crack during pregnancy, yet they continued to do it. The feelings of guilt increased rather than detered crack consumption. In addition, they did not desire to be pregnant through sex-for-crack exchange, yet no action was taken to prevent it from happening. It can be concluded that these women feel that they had little control over their life circumstances (Sharpe, 2001).

The importance of religion in determining the outcome of sex-for-crack pregnancies is also paradoxical. Abortion is considered "killing" by a majority of women who became pregnant; however, they continued to use drugs and exchange sex for crack while pregnant, placing the baby at risk for birth defects and/or sexually transmitted diseases (Sharpe, 2001).

Finally, the acceptance of a sex-for-crack–conceived pregnancy and the acceptance of the child into the family may be an indication that male disengagement from family life in this culture is nearly complete. Inner-city women have such low expectations for the men in their lives that the paternity of children may no longer be a major consideration.

In the next chapter, the lives of children conceived by sex for crack cocaine, mothering sex-for-crack children, and child neglect will be examined.

Chapter 8

Sex-for-Crack Children

Seventeen children conceived by sex for crack were discovered in the study. Sixteen were currently living. One child, a boy, died shortly after birth. His mother was Toni. The sex-for-crack children's ages ranged from 1 month to 17 years of age with a mean of 4.24 and standard deviation of 4.25. Most of these children were very young. The age of the oldest child gives a misleading impression of the distribution range. The next oldest child was age 9. Fourteen of the children (82.4 percent) were ages 6 and under. The mode of the distribution was age 1. Two children were less than 1 year old. Seven of the children were male and ten were female.

LIFE CIRCUMSTANCES
OF SEX-FOR-CRACK CHILDREN

Only five children were currently in the custody of their mothers. Seven children were cared for by their mother's relatives: three were in the custody of the maternal grandmothers and four children were cared for by other members of their mother's families. Two children were removed from their mother by the state of Georgia. One child was cared for by the paternal grandmother, and another child was legally adopted by a family not related to the mother.

Children who remained with their mothers were mostly very young. The seventeen-year-old's mother reported that he was in her custody, but this child was nearly a legal adult. The other four children living with their mothers were two years old or younger. The mothers of these young children managed to keep them because they were all undergoing drug treatment in a long-term, inpatient facility equipped with a nursery and day care center. This kind of treatment is extremely rare. The facility also sponsored a pregnant and postpartum women's program as well. Unfortunately, in 2004 this facility closed its doors due to lack of funding. Three of the five women who were pregnant by exchange when interviewed were participants in the program. The other two were on the streets and still actively using crack. Child care is a major obstacle for many crack-addicted women seeking recovery from drug use. Furthermore, most treatment facilities are not designed to care for pregnant addicts.

Five of the seventeen sex-for-crack children were fathered by drug dealers. Five of the children's fathers were unknown. Seven children were fathered by a casual acquaintance of their mother's.

CHILDREN'S RELATIONSHIPS
WITH FAMILY MEMBERS

The research participants were asked: "Are sex-for-crack–conceived children treated differently by family members?" Most women answered that question with "no!" One of my respondents, Sylvia, made that very clear:

My little baby, my four-month-old son, his father was a drug dealer. I decided to have the baby because his father and I became closer. He is in prison now for drug trafficking. . . . I don't believe in abortion. . . . My relatives don't know that the baby was conceived [in a sex-for-crack exchange]. . . . I think that he will be treated equally with my other children. . . . I love my baby. I am learning to be a mother because I was always able to throw them [her children] off on someone else. This time I am taking responsibility for myself. That's why I came into the [treatment] program. I didn't have a life, the life that I was living. Now I'm just like a newborn baby. I'm trying to learn how to live. I'm learning how to have patience with the child. . . . It will be difficult for me because a child needs two parents. . . . I really believe that he [the baby] is a blessing to me. My higher power seen to that.

Again, we see a reference to spirituality in conjunction with a sex-for-crack child. Sylvia's two older children were split between her mother and sister. The youngest baby was her opportunity to be a mother again. Sylvia's family was not aware of the circumstances of her baby's conception. In April's case, her family was fully aware that her son was conceived in a drug-sex trade. April talks about her baby:

I love him [the baby]. I am just a mother and he is my son, I guess. Ain't gon' be no difference. I don't have no kind of resentment [toward the baby], whatsoever. I love him just like the other ones. . . . They [my family] know [that he was conceived by sex for crack]. They say they still love him. It wasn't no shocker. . . .

Although most women reported that their sex-for-crack children were not treated differently by family members and friends, some women, under special circumstances, believed that their sex-for-crack children were treated differently. Valerie's mother was willing to take care of her older daughter, but distanced herself when Valerie became impregnated by a drug dealer. Valerie explains:

This [sex-for-crack pregnancy] happened one time. I had the baby. I had the baby because it wasn't the child's fault. I have custody. She is one year old. The drug dealer is her father. . . . I don't believe in abortions. I tried to have an abortion, but it didn't work out. Every place I was calling, they said I was too far along. The one place that said I wasn't too far along, but I didn't have transportation to get there. I just felt like God blesses us with things for a reason. I just couldn't see myself giving her up, the further along I got, knowing that it's a human inside of me, and just thinking what if my mother did me like that. I couldn't do it. . . . My family doesn't like it but it is nothing they can do about it.

I believe that she is treated differently. I feel like she is treated differently, 'Cause with my nine-year-old, my mother take her and let her live with her for four years. When I was pregnant with her [sex-for-crack baby] she wouldn't give me nowhere to stay. When I had the baby she [mother] didn't come to see me in the hospital. When I called her and told her that I had the baby and that it was a girl my mother said, "What you want me to do?" I just felt like I was getting put out with her. She didn't say that I know we had problems in the past, but let's try to work it out together. You can come stay with me but I'm only giving you a month or two weeks. She didn't do that. She just washed her hand of it and said I don't care where y'all go. I think she did that because of the things I did, but I don't think what I did should reflect on my kids. . . . I love her [one-year-old] to death. She got some of my temper and her father's temper. She has never been abused. She gets along, but she is a little feisty. She wants to take stuff from the other kids. She doesn't see her father because, from what I hear, he is incarcerated. . . . I feel close to her because with my nine-year-old, she had my whole family. But with me and her, we are alone. I went through a lot with her when I was pregnant. . . . I think it's hard for me to be a mother to any of my kids. Because as long as I am using [drugs] and I am not living the way I should.

This is a very telling quote. Valerie could not understand her mother's reluctance to accept her sex-for-crack baby. Although their relationship was strained due to Valerie's first two out-of-wedlock pregnancies, she fully expected to receive help from her mother, regardless of her crack use, prostitution, and subsequent sex-for-crack pregnancy.

Dena's mother also drew the line when she became pregnant with her second sex-for-crack child. Her mother has custody of Dena's two older boys and her three-year-old sex-for-crack conceived daughter. The fourth pregnancy pushed her mother to the breaking point. Dena speaks of her first sex-for-crack child and then her current pregnancy.

My mother knows [that the three-year-old was sex-for-crack conceived] and she said she didn't want to take care of no more babies. She said she was tired of the children. She wouldn't give them up. . . . They treat all the kids the same. I have a better relationship with her [three-year-old] than with my boys. She respect me more. I talk to her on the phone. She told me to bring her brother and some candy, m&m's. . . . She has asthma. She has special doctors. My sister babysits her while my mom is at work. . . . Whenever I'm around she comes to me. She knows I'm her mother. . . .

It was hard [to be a mother at first] because I was out there in the street. It was the crack. I was not responsible. . . . I am pregnant now. I really didn't handle the situation; I was too far gone. I am seven-and-a-half-months pregnant. I don't know who the father is. I waited too late [to have an abortion]. . . . My mom knows [that the pregnancy was conceived by sex for crack]. She told me to get my tubes tied. She said that I will have to take care of this baby. I think I'm ready. I'm learning to. . . . It was my plan to give it to my aunt, but I feel differently now. I feel like I can today. But when I first got pregnant, I knew that I wouldn't be able to. . . . I don't think he will be treated different.

Though unstated, Valerie and Dena indicated that their sex-for-crack children will be treated differently by their families linked to their family's unwillingness to take on the responsibility of another child. As the story relates, Dena planned to give custody of the child inside her womb to her aunt. The hidden message in this text is the women's expectations concerning the welfare of their children: they expect the extended family to absorb them. There appears to be a disconnect between having children and taking care of them. Most of the women witnessed their mothers shift parental responsibility to the previous generation. They entered parenthood with the same expectations and believed that their drug use or involvement in prostitution would make no difference in the acceptance of their children. Perhaps their mothers' involvement with alcohol or drugs is related to their expectations as well. The women may view crack use in the same way their mothers viewed alcohol use.

MOTHERING SEX-FOR-CRACK CHILDREN

Mothering sex-for-crack children is difficult for a majority of the women simply because they do not have custody of them. The status of mother for some is in name only. Moreover, a number of women have children divided between and among relatives and foster care. Having children in the custody of relatives makes it simpler to establish some kind of visiting schedule. Some women developed methods to stay in contact with their children and continue the drug-user lifestyle. One woman reported making sure she took a bath before she went to her relative's home to visit her children. Dena reported scheduling a rest day at a friend's house before she visited her children. Dena explains:

I was always in the street. . . . I started going over to my friend's house to rest up before I went to see my kids. I knew he would give me money.

Kathy has three sex-for-crack–conceived children. Her aunt has custody of her seven-year-old and six-year-old. Kathy has custody of the two-year-old. Recall that she also has three older children in the custody of her very elderly grandmother. Kathy managed to juggle her crack street life and keep up with her children's lives. She received a lot of help from her family.

Kathy describes her mothering style with the seven-year-old and the two-year-old. The story concerning the six-year-old appears in the "Abuse, Neglect, and Abandonment" section later in this chapter. The six-year-old was the child born in a crack house.

When I found out [I was pregnant], I said "God." But I constantly kept getting high. I don't want no abortion, I don't know who the daddy is. I didn't want to kill it because I don't believe in abortion. I was killing it anyway, by smoking. So I started putting myself in a rehab. My conscious started bothering me, so I went and had myself admitted, after five months of smoking, to the Boulevard rehab. I stayed cleaned for a while. But after I came out of the hospital, I wasn't even out three days, I went out on my mission again. So DFACS was fixing to take her. She didn't have cocaine in her system when she was born, thank God. My family knows [that she was conceived in a sex-for-crack exchange], but they love her. They used to talk about it. They said, "Why is you keep laying up getting these babies and you ain't taking care of them? If we wasn't around, these children [seven- and six-year-old] would be separated and apart from each other. You need to stop and think about what you're doing." . . .

I don't think she is treated differently. . . . We are crazy about each other. She know I am Mama. We talks and she love to stay up under me. That's my "boot" [affectionate term]. She want to know when she can come and stay with me. I talk to her every day on the phone. I calls her. I call my baby. We are very close. . . .

So far, she does not have any learning problems. She is smart. She has not been abused to my knowledge. . . . She is doing good in school. We don't get no complaints on her. The teacher, when I talk to my aunt, always has good things to say about her. She is a good listener. Except she had one problem when she was working with the alphabet, she had problems with the "W." She had problems counting money. It wasn't the alphabet, it was counting money. She doesn't know the difference between a dime and a nickel. I thought she should be able to know that stuff. So she may have a problem with that. She have a thing with money. She can't count no money. She knows the difference between paper dollars, five dollars, ten dollars, she know what that is. But when it come down to the change, she can't tell the difference between the dime, the nickel, and the pennies. . . .

She gets along with other children and people. I don't know who her father is. I feel close to her because I know she is mine. I carried her. In spite of my drug addiction, I would still go home and take a bath and cuddle with her.

Babies know that "love." I'd come in, kiss her, and play with her. I would sleep up under her and wouldn't let her out of my eye sight. I might be home for two or three days, but we bonded within those days that I'm there. I would constantly have her in my arms. . . .

Right now, it is hard for me to be a mother to her. I am trying to come off the stuff [crack] and I needs some time to get myself together so I can be able to help her do things or have the patience to spend quality time with her without trying to, say one minute, I'm spending time with her, and then the next thing you know, in my mind I'm thinking, okay, it's time for me to go and get a hit. Okay, let me put you aside right now. I'll be back. . . .

My whole family is in a house. My grandmother is sick right now. My aunt comes over every day. She got a job and a car. In the morning she have time to pick them up and drop them off at school. She gets off in time and pick them up from school. Then they stay over to her grandmama house until eight or nine o'clock at night. Then they go home and get their baths and go to sleep. Then they get back up and start their routine over again. I got pregnant with Terry [two-year-old], and I didn't have an abortion for the same reason. I don't know who her father is. . . . I couldn't get rid of it [baby]. . . . My family doesn't know [that she was conceived in sex-for-crack exchange]. . . .

She is treated differently by my children, my aunt, and my grandmother. They say, "How come you can take care of this one and not the other two?"

She is treated differently because she with me and the other ones [children] ain't. My grandmother loves her but has a little resentment toward her too. She say, "Why is she so special and you got two more, right here, in the same age group, not too far behind her, that you can't [take care of]." Then I told them that "I know that I couldn't dump her off on y'all. Y'all got all the rest of them." I had to take responsibility somewhere. It ain't like I ain't going to get them [other children]. I'm working on that now. . . .

Kathy made a conscious decision that she must take care of her youngest child. When I interviewed her, she was making every effort to stay clean and take care of her baby. She was in an inpatient drug treatment facility, in a pregnant and postpartum women's program. Her family did not understand why she suddenly decided to take care of her sixth child when she has five children in the custody of others. Only one woman reported that she would have difficulty parenting her sex-for-crack child.

Amy was very much affected by her mother's alcohol addiction and her rejection of her as a child and again as an adult. She was ashamed that she did not know the identity of her biological father. She did not desire a similar experience for her child, but her sex-for-crack pregnancy was conceived by one of several men she had had sex with at the time she became pregnant. Amy explains:

I know it is gonna be difficult for me because it won't be like this is "John's" baby, my high school sweetheart. I don't know who [fathered] this child . . . I know the part of me that is this child, but I won't know the part of him that is his father. It's almost like having half a stranger. His father, I don't know. All I know is that it was a trick.

ABUSE, NEGLECT, AND ABANDONMENT

Not one of the women reported that their sex-for-crack–conceived children were abused, neglected, or abandoned. However, most of the sex-for-crack–conceived children had had substantial crack exposure before birth. Only one child did not sustain substantial prenatal crack exposure: the child born at the very beginning of the crack era; the seventeen-year-old. The range of exposure in months was 1 to 9, the mode was 9 months, and the mean was 6.61 with a standard deviation of 2.91. Fourteen children had six months' exposure or more.

Though no reports of overt child abuse or neglect were uncovered in this research, several incidents of covert abuse and neglect were discovered. Several women reported using welfare funds and food stamps to purchase drugs, leaving the children home alone and neglecting to feed or bathe them.

Valerie reports her difficulties managing motherhood with her crack habit:

It is hard for me to stay focused. A lot of times, I'm real agitated and don't want to be bothered with my kids or bothered with humans, period. It's like I be off into space. You could ask me a question and I be looking at you and don't hear nothing you be saying. . . . I couldn't manage being a good mother. Any money I got, if it wasn't but two or three dollars, I tried to find somebody that had money to put in with me to get a bag. Then I would leave my kids in the house to walk up the street.

Kathy conveys her lack of mothering abilities after becoming addicted to crack:

I got to the point where I didn't want to do them things [care for her children] no more. Those things weren't important to me anymore. The only thing I cared about was getting that next high. My kids was not important. Going to the movies was not important. Cooking dinner for them was not important. Taking their baths was not important. When they got sick, somebody else had to take them [to the doctor], because it wasn't important. Crack was important.

April reports her difficulties balancing motherhood and crack use. She also describes his sister's experiences mothering on crack and relates an episode when she really disappointed her children:

Crack made me lose them. When I had them, I didn't want to get up in the morning to take them to school. Because most of the time, I had been up all night, getting high. I didn't want to iron their clothes. It was really stupid. My son would tell me in a minute, "Mama, you didn't iron my pants right." I said, "You better wear them like that." That was terrible. . . .

I waited until they went to sleep to do crack 'cause I didn't want to embarrass them by seeing me high. They knew what it was, because they been around it all their lives. My son said, "Mama, you high." My fifteen-year-old would say, "Mama, why you keep getting geeked up? What's wrong with you? Do you need some help or something?" It used to make me feel so bad, knowing he knew. My daughter would sit there and shake her head. . . .

My sister didn't manage being a good mom at all. She sent her kids to school with half-dry clothes, dirty. Didn't have no socks on. No strings in the tennis shoes. . . . Let me tell you how I did my son one time. He was working for the

Olympics. He worked for two weeks and got paid. He was just bragging about what he was going to buy. I waited until he went to sleep and took all his money and smoked it. I felt like killing myself. He was crying. He asked me how could I do something like that. That same Christmas, I didn't buy my twelve-year-old nothing for Christmas. I was so sick on that shit. I would wrassle my daughter to the ground to take back money that I gave her so I could buy crack. What kind of mother is that? I wish I hadn't done that to my kids. I wish I had my kids back.

April's story shares vital information regarding the experience of children of crack-addicted mothers. These children are subjected to their mother's erratic behaviors and traumatized by instability in the home environment. April's impression of being a good mother simply meant that she was better at being a mother than her sister Carrie. (Recall Carrie's escapades from Chapter 5.) However, April's children were frustrated and bewildered at her behaviors. Imagine her fifteen-year-old son's disappointment when he found his mother had used his hard-earned money to purchase drugs. Imagine April's daughter's frustration with her mother wrestling money from her hand, and the disappointment a twelve-year-old child would have receiving nothing for Christmas. Now imagine these children in a public school classroom. The public school system cannot possibly meet the complex needs of children with home situations such as these.

The preceding stories suggest that children in the homes of crack-addicted mothers, whether sex-for-crack conceived or not, receive far less than adequate nurturing and discipline. It is unrealistic to expect children with this kind of background to be prepared for the demands of the education system without major initiatives to provide them with social and academic learning skills in the earliest years of schooling and long-term support from a committed mentoring program. One of the neglected dimensions in the investigation of the failure of public education in poor urban neighborhoods is the lack of consideration for marginalized children's home environment. Children's education should involve a strong partnership between the parents and the school. Ideally, during the first five years of a child's life, a significant amount of learning should occur at home. By the time a child is ready for kindergarten, he or she should have basic social and academic skills. In addition, when the formal learning process begins, the parent should support the educational efforts at school by monitoring school progress and ensuring that the child completes assignments on time and has the tools required for specific activities.

However, if a child has received almost no social or academic home training in the first five years of his or her life, it is unrealistic to expect a kindergarten teacher to correct the behavior problems that stem from deeply rooted emotional trauma at home in addition to teaching the child to read, write, and count. Furthermore, the strain of teaching children who approach the school environment unprepared to learn hampers the learning of children who are prepared to learn. Herein lies the dilemma of the public education system in many inner cities.

Raising children requires a kind of stability difficult for crack-addicted women to achieve. In the analyzed sample of women, covert child neglect occurred in a number of forms: use of family moneys for drugs, inadequate care and feeding, leaving children home alone, and disappointing the children during holidays.

The most graphic form of child abuse uncovered by this research was the use of crack cocaine during the delivery of a child and the birth of a child in a crack house. Two women, Kathy and April, reported using crack while in labor. Kathy relates the incident in which her second sex-for-crack baby was delivered in a crack house.

I didn't have not choice but to keep her. She didn't ask to be here. I don't believe in abortions. . . . I'm sure my family knows [that she was conceived in a sex-for-crack exchange], because I was walking the streets a lot when I got pregnant. They have made comments, "Well, do you know who this daddy is of this baby?" They say that I should be ashamed of myself. . . .

She is treated different because I messed her up. She is sick. I smoked the longest [when pregnant] with her. Her lungs is messed up. She's got asthma real bad. You have to have a machine [probably a nebulizer]. My aunt never leaves the house without it, because in case she have an asthma attack. She has to hook that machine and give her medicine through that. . . . She gets a lot of attention. . . .

I was eight months' pregnant. I found forty or fifty dollars on the ground. I wanted me a hit real bad. I was walking around watching people geeking. I had done had a taste earlier and it wasn't enough. I was real frustrated. I looked on the ground and there go some money, two twenties and a ten. The dope house was right across the street. I broke my neck getting over there. I bought four, four dimes. I had ten dollars left. I took it and went in the house and my grandma locked the burglar bars. It had to be about twelve thirty or one o'clock in the morning. I went in there and she locked the burglar bar door. I sat down in the rocking chair in my room. I started dropping them [the rocks] on [the straight shooter] whole. And they were some big ones. I dropped them in whole, I was inhaling, holding in the smoke and all of a sudden, my stomach started hurting. That wasn't enough. It was really hurting that I had to stop. I put it down for a minute and I got to twisting and turning. I was high. Only thing I know was that I still got my dope and I was fin' to keep smoking. And I'm steady dropping them on. After I finished all four of them bags still had plenty left in my shooter. I finished that up. I knew I was hurting. I said, "Oh, Grandmama, I'm hurting." Grandma said, "I'm not fin' to let you out of this house. This don't make no damn sense!" I said, "Grandmama, please let me out!" She eventually gave my daughter the key and she let me out. By the time I made it down to the steps, I felt pressure coming through my pants. It was my baby's head, already. I was wet and I didn't pay that no attention. But the head was already there. The pants was holding her in there. So I walked wide legged all the way back across the street to the dope house. I was standing there with my legs wide open and I kept feeling more pressure. It got worse. I was handing him [the dope dealer] the money, and all of a sudden, I just had to start pulling down my pants. He [dope dealer] said, "Oh no, what are you doing?" I said, "Just move out of the way. My baby is coming; my baby is coming." So the next thing you know, everybody [in the dope house] left me in there. So I took my pants off. I had to hold her head and I just pulled her on out. Then they [paramedics] came. They put her on the machine then. They took me to the hospital.

She had traces of crack cocaine [in her system]. DFACS was going to keep her. They wasn't gon' release her to me in the hospital. So, here I go again, I called my aunt, crying, "Come and get my baby; they won't give her to me." My aunt was there for me again. . . .

She weighed six pounds when she was born. She has asthma real bad. She can't run around like normal children. After a while, you have to make her sit down. She stay sick a lot too. She run fevers constantly. She gets in moods where she just lays around and don't want to be bothered. . . . She is crazy about me. She knows that I'm Mama. She doesn't have any emotional problems or learning disabilities, or physical handicaps. . . . She is doing great in school. The teacher says she needs to be an actress. They say she is good. When they have plays and stuff, the children sing songs, you can't hear nobody but her. She ain't scared of the stage or the people out there watching or nothing. She gets along with people. I don't know who her father is. . . . She is special because, there are so many reasons that she is special. Number one, because I carried her; she came out of me. And I nearly killed her. That makes her even more special, she hung in there, she didn't come out with so and so and so, and she made it through. It is not hard to be a mother to her.

Kathy had tremendous guilt about this pregnancy, this child, and her relationship with her. In order to cope with her actions she rationalized that, in spite of the circumstances of her birth in a crack house, the six-year-old was doing well in school and was free of learning and physical disabilities. However, the child had asthma and required breathing treatments. Kathy admits that this particular child is special simply because she survived long-term exposure to crack in the womb and birth under unimaginable circumstances.

The findings concerning mothering sex-for-crack children did not vary significantly from other studies conducted on the subject of mothers who use crack cocaine (Kearney et al., 1994a,b; Pursley-Crotteau and Stern, 1996). The women in the study valued the status of motherhood and strongly identified with being a mother. They used the same parenting strategies with their sex-for-crack–conceived children as with their other children. Furthermore, most women (eighteen) felt that it would not be more difficult to parent their sex-for-crack children than it was to parent the others. Similar to findings of Kearney and colleagues (1994b), the women in this study made efforts to separate their crack-user roles from their motherhood roles. In fact, one could argue that the women lived double lives.

Leading double lives was possible for most because they did not have custody of their children. The status of mother for some was in name only. As with their other children, sex-for-crack children were generally cared for by someone else. These children received high levels of drug exposure before birth. Most of the children were accepted by the women's families, but at least two were not. The women devised special methods to maintain contact with their children and continued to use crack. However, most reported that mothering on crack was nearly impossible. Their children were neglected and at times left at home with no adult supervision. Using crack cocaine up to the very point of delivery was one of the most startling findings of this research. This phenomenon demonstrates the powerfully addictive nature of the drug and supports Robert Staples' (1991c) theory that crack addiction contributed to the death of black motherhood in poor communities.

Chapter 9 presents a synthesis of the findings and links them to the social and economic forms described in Chapter 1. The influences on sex-for-crack pregnancies are considered with respect to the difficult conditions present in the women's lives. Implications suggesting that motherhood and fatherhood in this context have changed are presented. Policy recommendations are suggested for drug treatment and for child welfare.

Chapter 9

Discussion, Conclusions, and Policy Suggestions

DISCUSSION

Poverty, substance use, teenage pregnancy, and single-parenthood are not issues unique to only blacks in America; they are pervasive among other racial ethnic groups in America and pervasive all over the world. However, in the United States, with institutionalized constraints on economic opportunities; limited access to employment systems; declining federal-income transfer and job-training programs; and tax-based, elite-favoring school systems, the aforementioned issues complicate an already complicated existence that many blacks, especially women, must endure and overcome to achieve even marginal self-sufficiency.

By the 1980s, inner-city poor neighborhoods were at a low point. The introduction of crack cocaine set these struggling communities on an even more destructive path. Crack cocaine cannot be blamed for all of the problems in poor black neighborhoods, but surely it is the single entity that very quickly made bad conditions much worse. Using crack, exchanging sex for crack, and the consequences of these actions add additional barriers to gaining a niche in mainstream life.

The combination of a sexualized image of poor black women, strained relationships between unemployed black men and women, and widespread poverty all contributed to the development of the sex-for-crack cocaine barter system. This system places women at an extreme disadvantage for a number of reasons. The women in this study routinely engaged in unprotected sex for crack with a variety of males from all walks of life, including men in their neighborhoods, strangers passing through town, and drug dealers. Women who exchange sex for crack are at risk for contracting HIV infection and becoming pregnant by prostitution clients.

Centers for Disease Control and Prevention (2005) statistics indicate that the rate of HIV infection is sixteen times higher in black women compared with white women. Black women accounted for 64 percent of HIV infections reported in 2003. AIDS is now the leading cause of death for black women ages eighteen to thirty-four (Centers for Disease Control and Prevention, 2005). Race/ethnicity itself does not contribute to contracting HIV infection. However, strong correlates of HIV infection include poverty, illegal substance use, and sexually transmitted diseases. As described in Chapter 1, pervasive structural and geographically concentrated poverty in the form of fewer breadwinner jobs, collapsing infrastructure, and emigration of the working and middle classes opened windows of opportunity for the crack economy to absorb unemployed, marginalized men and transform entire neighborhoods into crack production, distribution, and consumption centers. The crack infrastructure evolved to replace the void in economic opportunities, and became the major employer in poor neighborhoods. As described in Chapters 5 and 6, women were introduced to crack during social gatherings, by men during romantic encounters, or by friends or family. Women who had access to public transfer funds became the primary crack consumers. Crack addiction influences many women to engage in unsafe sexual practices and inconsistent use of condoms, placing them at risk for contracting sexually transmitted diseases, including HIV. Contracting sexually transmitted diseases increases the likelihood of contracting HIV infection through open genital lesions.

Of the forty-six women screened, seven (15 percent) reported HIV-positive status. Regarding another consequence of sex-for-crack exchange, half of the screening sample of women who exchanged sex for crack became pregnant through one or more of those exchanges. Of the first eight women screened, five had become pregnant by exchange. After thirty-four women were identified, eighteen reported having become pregnant by exchange. When forty-four poor black female crack users who exchanged sex for crack were located, twenty-one had at one time become pregnant by exchange. Thus, in this analysis, nearly 50 percent of the women who exchanged sex for crack became pregnant at least once. Furthermore, roughly 25 percent became pregnant by exchange more than once. In addition, 41.4 percent of the pregnancies resulted in live births, 17.1 percent resulted in miscarriages, 17.1 percent resulted in abortions, 7.3 percent in tubal pregnancies, 4.9 percent in stillbirths, and 12.2 percent of the women were pregnant when interviewed. Thus, it can be argued that sex-for-crack exchange influences reproductive outcomes in the forms of unplanned pregnancies, unwanted children, multiple abortions, and miscarriages among poor black female crack users.

The neighborhoods of the study participants may feel the repercussions of these pregnancies by the increased number of neglected children in their communities. Many men who hire these women for prostitution services leave the inner city without any sense of responsibility toward any conceptions that may have occurred. Furthermore, the men in their communities have been given a new weapon with which to control them. Crack has given unearned and illegitimate power to many poor black men. The women fight back in the ways they are able to, but the ultimate victor is the one who holds the crack sacks. The majority of the time, it is men who control the distribution of crack.

SEX-FOR-CRACK PREGNANCIES
AND THEIR OUTCOMES

Severity of crack use exerted the most pressure on all pregnancy outcomes. The cultural factors that also influenced the women's decisions about sex-for-crack pregnancies were counterbalanced heavily by severe crack use. In fact, crack use disabled most women and held them captive from all logical thought. They became high again and again—even after it was clear a child was conceived. Religious beliefs and the social-organization patterns, which emphasize female gender role primacy in families, were found to influence pregnancy outcomes as well; however, these influences were greatly overshadowed by the extremely addictive power of crack and its induced mental paralysis. Severity of crack use was found to influence women to have abortions: the women who had abortions did so in order to keep getting high. However, having the strength to stop using crack long enough to go to an abortion clinic was directly related to the relative severity of crack use. When women were in or near the beginning of their addiction and the crack compulsion had not completely dominated their lives, the commitment to maintain the crack-user role took the form of an active approach. In other words, if they became pregnant and desired to continue using crack, they actively sought an abortion to alleviate themselves of the responsibility of having a child.

Women who were more deeply addicted to crack were also committed to maintaining the user role, but they passively continued to use crack after a pregnancy was detected and ignored the situation until it became too late to safely abort the pregnancy. Especially explanatory were the accounts from women who aborted sex-for-crack pregnancies early in their drug-use history and later gave birth to a sex-for-crack–conceived child as the addiction deepened. As the crack compulsions grew stronger, it was more difficult to break free from the geek-and-freak cycle long enough to have an abortion.

As mentioned, another cultural dimension found influential in the process of pregnancy outcomes was religion. All of the women expressed deep religious beliefs, but their beliefs were paradoxical in nature. On one hand, they believed in God and his protection for them. On the other hand, they did not apply the values or principles normally associated with their self-identified Christian denominations to their lives. Many women expressed a religion-inspired aversion to abortion, but these same women used crack for their entire pregnancies involving sex-for-crack children and some of their other children as well. Furthermore, women who had abortions considered themselves deeply spiritual as well. Religious beliefs were largely symbolic and not prescriptions for behavior. The women harbored values and ideals that their lives could not fulfill, and even then their beliefs were tempered by the severe level of crack consumption.

The social organization of poor black communities, which shifted toward minimal male responsibility in their biological children's lives, exerted indirect pressure on the pregnancy outcomes. This pressure was experienced as an acceptance of the children after they were born. Some women acknowledged that though, in theory, a child should have two parents, most women had not experienced the presence of a father role model in their lives and did not know what to expect of a good father for their children. Here again we find disparity between values and reality. Moreover, marriage is so uncommon among inner-city poor blacks that it is no longer an institutional basis for family formation. In addition, any form of pair bonding is not required for the production of children.

Though the women were ambiguous about their conceptions in the context of prostitution, sex-for-crack children were valued as members of their mothers' families. However, the children are only valued after they are born. As the babies remain unseen in the womb, the women continue to use crack in significant proportions without regard for the children's prenatal development. Valuing the children after they arrive has no influence over the women continuing drug use while they are pregnant. In this light, social influence is only peripheral to pregnancy outcome. The prominent social-organization structure influences the acceptance of a sex-for-crack–conceived child after his or her birth, and his or her disregard while in the womb.

As described earlier, some women desired to have abortions but declined to obtain them directly due to severe crack consumption. Others simply increased crack use to avoid or deny the presence of the pregnancies. Crack-use severity is by far the most influential agent in determining pregnancy outcomes. The commitment to continue crack use was strong for all women. The women who used crack at a lesser degree took an active role in preserving their ability to use crack without the complications a child would bring by having abortions. The passive women, caught in the throes of extremely severe geeking and freaking, simply let the pregnancies develop without interference or prenatal care.

Regardless of whether they aborted a child, religious beliefs were present for all respondents in the qualitative component of the study. Crack-use severity pushed through their religious beliefs with different outcomes. After the child is born, the women accept him or her, distance themselves from the conception, and minimize the importance of the child's father. Therefore, a social-organization structure that stresses female gender role primacy and perpetuates male disengagement from families of procreation influences the outcomes of sex-for-crack pregnancies in indirect ways. The crack addiction shapes the women's individual responses to cultural influences as well.

AWARENESS OF RISK

Cognitive awareness of the risk of pregnancy while engaging in unprotected sex for crack is complex. The women's backgrounds played a significant role in constructing the parameters for sexual risk taking. Early in the women's lives their sexuality was coped with by avoiding it. Some women were not informed about their bodies in time to avoid humiliation, embarrassment, and confusion when they reached sexual maturity and began menstruating. Failing to receive vital information about sex and reproduction rendered the women vulnerable to coerced sexual activities without full knowledge of what was happening to them. The role of early and comprehensive sex education for this particular demographic group cannot be overemphasized. Knowledge is truly power in this case. As can be seen from their experiences, lack of knowledge left them powerless. The legacy of powerlessness over their sexuality and reproductive potential causes a perception of powerlessness over avoiding pregnancy.

The findings in this study support other studies on crack users and condom use. Crack users rarely use condoms when engaging in risky sexual acts. This study suggests explanations for why the women do not use condoms to protect themselves from sexually transmitted diseases and unplanned pregnancies. According to the study participants, the powerful desire for obtaining crack leads them to expose themselves to possible pregnancy or even AIDS. Underlying the crack motivation is the legacy of powerlessness in confronting the realities and consequences of sexuality. The women mentally disconnect prostitution sex from conceptions. They engage in unprotected vaginal sex with tricks and give little thought to the possibility that they might become pregnant. When pregnancies occur, many of the women invoke the spirit of God into their evaluation of the pregnancy.

It is important to note that fifteen out of the nineteen women who participated in the ethnographic interviews believed that babies were conceived by God. Many women felt that their sex-for-crack children were sent to them by God. This supports the findings of Kearney et al. (1994a). Kearney and colleagues' study of sex and fertility during crack use suggests that poor black female crack users who become pregnant view their pregnancies as gifts from God rather than chosen responsibilities. Several women in the present study thought they would not have become pregnant if God had not ordained it.

Religious beliefs play a role in the willingness to take sexual risks and in the acceptance of the results of the risk taking. In some ways, the women are trapped by their religious beliefs. They accept their conceptions as a gift from God, but use crack to medicate their feelings of ambivalence toward the pregnancy. Once again the symbolism of religion and not religion can be seen as a motivation to behavior change.

Powerlessness is a recurrent theme in this analysis. The women are not empowered to take control over their reproductive potential and outcomes, whether sex-for-crack conceived or otherwise. Sex and babies simply happen for these women, and, for the most part, are not conscious decisions or life choices. Before using crack, most women became sexually active without empowerment over their bodies. After becoming addicted to crack, the powerlessness over their bodies continued, but with exposure to more numerous partners, thereby increasing sexual risk.

Figuring heavily in the cognitive perception of risk are numerous inaccuracies about the facts of reproduction. The answers to the true-false sex-knowledge questions were very revealing. A majority of the women believed that coitus interruptus prevents pregnancy. A number of women believed other inaccuracies about human reproduction. Furthermore, the open-ended questions revealed that some women relied on street myths about the likelihood of pregnancy for crack-using females.

Some women thought that drug use made women less fertile, and at least one woman believed douches could prevent pregnancies. These examples point to lack of knowledge about sex and reproduction in adulthood as well as in childhood. Although cocaine use has been shown to make women's menstrual cycles more irregular, most women remain able to conceive babies if there are not other health issues present that decrease fertility. Irregular cycles may mislead the women into falsely assuming that they cannot become pregnant. A woman's history of irregular cycles while addicted to crack may play a role in the initial denial of sex-for-crack pregnancies. The combination of poor knowledge about sex and reproduction with crack addiction functions to exacerbate sexual risk taking.

CHILD LOSS AND CUSTODY ISSUES

Child loss was a common experience for the women. Some women lost custody of their children as a result of early motherhood. Eight women had become pregnant as teenagers. Some gave custody of their children to relatives because they were too young to care for them. The results suggest that motherhood for poor black women is at a critical juncture. For several generations, the responsibilities associated with motherhood have shifted to the previous generation. Teenage pregnancy was a principal occurrence in this phenomenon. In the recent past, poor black women have borne the sole responsibility of raising children. More recently it appears that the women are no longer willing to shoulder the responsibility, and if there is no extended family in place, the children are left with no one to care for them. Crack has given them the ability to first mentally disengage, and, when the addiction takes over, the women then physically disengage. With widespread crack use among women, the loopholes in the extended family have widened.

The shortened years between generations caused by teen pregnancy and prolific crack use leading to sexual risk taking has overwhelmed extended families by flooding communities with very young children. The reservoir of stable, older adults cannot keep up with the influx of these children. For the crack users in this study, a disconnect exists between having children and raising them. The women fully expect the extended family system to support any children they may produce, because they have failed to recognize that this system has been overwhelmed by the sheer numbers of children requiring homes. It is not that women are having more children due to crack. It is simply that fewer women are taking care of their own children. In a sense, the women are responding to parenting the same way many of their mothers responded. When their mothers were unable to care for them, the women were pushed to various relatives' homes. The women in the study approach parenting with the same expectations. Many expected others to take care of their children. But with an increase in poverty and drug addiction in inner cities there are fewer stable families or even stable individuals willing to take on the responsibility.

When children are raised with confusing home lives and are ambiguously placed with relatives who may be reluctant to take them, they frequently repeat the behaviors of their parents and the cycle begins again. As more poor black mothers on crack abandon their children, their grasp on the legendary self-sacrificial black motherhood referred to so often in the literature and in the popular culture, slips further away.

CRACK USE, MOTHERHOOD, AND OPPORTUNITY STRUCTURE

Robert Staples (1994) suggests that crack has caused the death of poor black motherhood. In contrast, this book offers that poor black motherhood was damaged first by structural changes and the decline of pair bonding for the stability of children. These changes predate crack's introduction by twenty or more years. When millions of young black girls became pregnant out of wedlock and had babies in the 1970s, the legitimization of male disengagement from the responsibility of their offspring began. The increased pressure on the extended family began then as well. This generation of children was transferred into the care of grandmothers and aunts as their mothers tried to finish school or find work. The children accepted the single-parent, female-headed families as the norm, because these were the families they witnessed growing up. When they returned to the care of their mothers and reached sexual maturity, they were often left at home alone while their mothers worked to support them. Their peer groups became extremely important support systems for them. This led to early sexual experimentation and pregnancy, drug and alcohol use, and criminal activities. Variations on this theme were heard over and over again from the women who participated in the qualitative interviews. The women repeated the pattern established by their mothers and had children before they finished school or were employed. Early parenthood interfered with achievement of the skills necessary to participate in all but the lowest service-sector jobs.

This study is not a moral indictment against teenage pregnancy nor is it a value judgment against out-of-wedlock conceptions. Rather, this is an analysis of the structure of opportunity and life chances in the American economy of the twenty-first century. The bifurcated structure of the economy and the complexities of hiring practices requires a solid education and determination in order to find a job in the face of numerous obstacles. Low-paying service jobs are always in demand, as are high-paying technical positions. For most other jobs, the bureaucratic barriers, hidden job markets, inadequate contingencies in automated telephone job information lines, and poorly trained personnel staffs so prevalent in the employment scene today discourage all but the most tenacious job seekers. In addition to having marketable skills, one must also have a particular savvy in self-marketing.

Poor black women who have dropped out of school face even more barriers than do educated women. Without education and intimate knowledge of how the politics of getting a job are played, poor black women have few chances of obtaining a life-sustaining job. One of the best ways to be left out of the competitive job market is to drop out of school. It appears that inner-city poor blacks are currently in a downward spiral linked to increasingly younger women with a higher degree of unpreparedness who are becoming mothers. Motherhood for the women in this analysis was largely symbolic. The day-to-day actions that define motherhood were out of their level of experience. Several women felt encouraged that their children acknowledged them as "mother." It was important for them to be acknowledged as mother even if they did not actually function in the roles of mothering. This is reminiscent of the absent fathers discussed in Chapter 2. One woman in particular indicated that her daughter knew that she was the mother and thus asked for m&m's on her next visit. Motherhood remains an important title for self-definition, but the criteria for being a good mother were often obscure due to inadequate exposure to a role model. Lack of a role model is often cited as a problem for poor black male youth. The findings of this study suggest that female youth suffer from this same disadvantage.

LIFE QUALITY OF SEX-FOR-CRACK CHILDREN

The lives of the sex-for-crack children did not vary significantly from the women's other children. Most of the sex-for-crack children in this analysis did not live with their mothers. This was true of their other children as well. The legacy of custody transference was very evident. Only five of the living sixteen sex-for-crack children were in their mothers' care. A number of the women's children were divided among various relatives, in adoptive homes, or in foster care. All but one of the sex-for-crack children were born exposed to crack. Many of the women's other children were born exposed to the drug as well.

A sex-for-crack child's status in the family was dependent upon circumstances, birth order, and, most important, the relationship between the child's mother and her family. If the mother's relationship with her mother or other relatives was strained, there was more resentment and reluctance to take responsibility for the child. Birth order was also a factor in the family acceptance of the sex-for-crack child. Families were generally willing to care for one or two of the women's children, but some family members balked at the responsibility of taking care of additional children as the women continued to become pregnant.

Several women attempted to reaffirm motherhood status by retaining custody of their youngest sex-for-crack child. Although their older children were cared for by relatives, two of the women in the study sought treatment in order to keep their youngest children. The women's tenacity at holding on to the youngest child was evaluated with dismay and confusion in their families. Members of the family responded with questions about the women's lack of dedication to the older children. So, a sex-for-crack child born under these circumstances may be treated differently by the family due to his or her mother's special attention. This differential treatment could be detrimental to the child later in life. The children cared for by others may feel rejected or abandoned by their mothers, and may question why their mother chose to keep the youngest child and not them.

Eighteen of the nineteen women in the study felt that it would not be difficult to mother their sex-for-crack children. All, however, stressed that it was difficult to function as a mother while addicted to crack. Motherhood was problematic since most of their sex-for-crack and other children were not currently living with them. Several women expressed gratitude that their families had custody of their children and that visits were possible. The life of a crack user and any attempts at mothering were compartmentalized by many women. Going "home" to visit the children was balanced with leaving home to pursue crack use. These two facets of life were maintained separately for most.

The women understood the dangerous lives in the crack world and desired to protect their children from it. Their families (mothers, grandmothers, aunts, cousins) to some extent enabled them to lead double lives. Extended families allowed the women to be involved with their children intermittently—coming off the street to rest for a few days and then returning to the days and nights of geeking and freaking.

According to their mothers, the sex-for-crack children in this analysis were not victims of abuse, at least after birth. This claim can be debated. The abuse the children suffered before they were born, in some cases right up to the moment of birth, affected them after birth as well. The findings suggest that crack use during pregnancy is not unusual in the crack world. The empirical and anecdotal evidence from the women point to notable crack use during pregnancy. After birth, if children remain with their mothers, the disorganized life of a crack user is often more devastating than prenatal drug exposure. Child neglect was very common in this analysis, and neglect can be considered a form of abuse.

In poor families, resources are so scarce that every dollar is a significant part of the income. Purchasing crack drains the meager money the women obtain from welfare or work. A number of the women reported using the money that was intended to buy food for their children to buy drugs instead. Furthermore, children were sometimes left home alone while their mothers went to purchase crack. Incidents of this kind of neglect underlie loss of custody for many. When family members or the child welfare representatives discovered that the children were living in apartments with no food in the refrigerator or were being left home alone, they intervened and removed the children from the mother's custody.

Two of the most powerful findings of the present study is the birth of a child in a crack house and the report of another woman who continued to use crack while she was in labor. These incidents are graphic reminders of the power of crack to influence behavior. Having a baby in a crack house is detrimental to the health of the woman and the child. Crack houses are unsanitary places with dangerous people about. Eight months pregnant, Kathy embarked on a crack binge, and even though she was in labor she could not resist going to the crack house to get one more hit of crack. This report was the highest degree of child abuse in the study. Furthermore, Kathy was not the only woman in this analysis who reported smoking crack during labor. It is hard to imagine what could possibly motivate a woman in labor to continue drug use when her child is about to be born.

The answer may lie in the chemical compound produced when crack is burned: methylecgonidine (MEG). The body of research described in the literature review concerning MEG, the crack pyrolysis product, points to the potential for unknown biological and behavioral consequences of ingesting this chemical. Moreover, the long-term effects to the heart and lungs after MEG exposure raises many questions about its potential long-term effects on behavior. The evidence that MEG has the ability to bond with substances in the body, perhaps brain chemicals, indicates a need for further research. To be sure, crack addiction changes behavior, as the women in the study have shown.

Crack use during gestation and the child neglect patterns described earlier are evidence that the drug changes behavior patterns. The inability to discontinue crack use during labor demonstrates that the drug has the potential to alter thought processes much more than commonly believed.

DISCUSSION OF RELATED ISSUES

The findings regarding the lives of the women presented in Chapters 5-8 suggest two other points for discussion: (1) reevaluation of the effectiveness of the extended family among extremely poor blacks, and (2) tension between poor black men and women.

First, the extent to which the extended family has been impacted by severe economic pressures, change and dislocation, and shifts in opportunity structures is an area requiring further research. In the literature, the extended family among blacks is touted as a safety valve for the stability of families. The studies cited were conducted in the 1960s and early 1970s, before the full impact of American economic transition was felt. Additional research is required for the evaluation of the impact of these processes in current inner-city life. The extended family system failed to protect and nurture a notable number of women in this study. When their mothers were unable to care for them, they were pushed to various relatives' homes. Their extended families did not provide the women with adequate role models for motherhood. Furthermore, the early lives of the women point to inadequate nurturing and adult supervision.

The women in the study approach parenting with similar standards. They expect others to take care of their children. However, community structures have changed so much in recent years that these expectations are often unrealized. The weak extended family has become even weaker due to the prevalence of crack. As well, the combination of structural constraints and a change in sexual codes has severely decreased the prevalence of marriage among poor black people.

Second, tension between poor black males and females has reached a high point. Marriage as a partnership for the pooling of resources and skills and for the nurturing of children has been abandoned in inner cities. Poor black men and women spend significant portions of their lives without partners. This places them in an extended dating mode. All of the women in the ethnographic portion of the study could not get beyond this part of life, and this contributed to the prevalence of exchanging sex for crack among poor black women. Recall that forty-six out of fifty-two poor black female crack users reported exchanging sex for crack. The trend away from pair bonding has created a failure to move forward in the family life cycle. Men and women are constantly moving from one relationship to another. Children may be produced, but the relationships that produce them are relatively short lived. As the results show, serial relationships and changing household compositions confuse children and leave them open for neglect and isolation. Any mainstream single mother knows that trying to raise children and manage a love life can be stressful and overwhelming. However, mainstream women have other sources of support that can buffer the combination of stressors. For poor black men and women, searching for a mate can be a lifelong process.

Pair bonding may have less importance for raising children in affluent families. Current debates exist on both sides of this issue. It can be argued that families with abundant resources can, to some extent, compensate for a missing partner. In poor black communities, the strength of pair bonding sustained families though manumission and segregation. Single parenthood did not become the dominant family pattern until late in the twentieth century.

A paradox of single parenthood in this context is that the men expect the women to be good mothers without their support. Furthermore, in the crack culture, male drug dealers sell drugs to women, and often sell drugs to pregnant women, yet the women are derided for their actions and not the men. The new dynamics of gender relations and the shift away from resource sharing in bonded pairs among poor black men and women is another topic for further research.

SOCIAL STRUCTURE AND THE LEGACY
OF SOCIAL CHANGE

Black social and familial structures in America have weathered a number of historic upheavals. Social and family structures have been weakened, but not eliminated, by slavery, the sharecropping system, segregation, and by the unforeseen consequences of desegregation. The United States' schizophrenic public policy toward blacks has reaped what it has sown throughout the course of the country's existence. Shifting with the political tide, the United States has been able to provide access to achieving the American dream for only some black Americans, leaving a large pool of men, women, and children circling the perimeter of opportunities, left largely outside.

The social structures present in inner cities, damaged by historic consequences, were rapidly superimposed by the crack cocaine social and economic structure. The sex-for-crack barter system quickly followed, and as a result, roles for men and women changed. The findings suggest that gender roles are in a state of transition for poor, inner-city blacks, and more important, that the meaning of motherhood and fatherhood may have changed due to crack use.

In the past, clearer definitions of the responsibilities of motherhood existed for poor black women. Moreover, women formerly assumed breadwinner as well as supportive roles in their families. Crack cocaine's introduction to inner cities has altered social structures and economic processes, causing many poor black women to lose the social prominence they once held. Crack dealers simply show up in neighborhoods when the welfare checks arrive, and are assured of harvesting that bounty. Without the money to support their families, the women in the study were unable to function in the instrumental role of female head of household. Furthermore, women who exchanged sex for crack, became pregnant, and gave birth generally did so without any support from the man who fathered the child. In most instances the woman did not know who fathered the child. The results also demonstrate that the women in the study used drugs during a significant portion of their pregnancies. How did crack cocaine addiction weaken motherhood and its traditional responsibilities so quickly? Where were the stabilizing social forces to resist these changes?

The explanation offered here is that the strength of social roles depends on the strength of the social structure. A weak social structure produces weakened social roles. These weakened roles are then vulnerable to rapid change from outside forces that the weak social structure cannot stop. In turn, the ambiguity of social roles and responsibilities weakens the fabric of the social structure. As reported previously, long before using crack, the women in the study were struggling with a variety of life's challenges in a number of areas: parents' substance abuse, truncated education opportunities, limited access to jobs, and difficult relationships with men. Furthermore, the data showed that their families of origin had their share of difficulties also. Inadequate role modeling for motherhood was also apparent. These conditions provided little resistance to the involvement with crack or to the involvement in exchanging sex for crack. The findings suggest that a strong and stable social structure is essential for stability in social roles.

Furthermore, with consistent damage to black family and social structures occurring during every subsequent social reorganization coupled with the oscillating doors of economic opportunity, the poorest black families have borne the fullest impact of discriminatory practices, and, at present, have been all but abandoned by America at large. Indeed, policymakers, instead of following history and giving consideration to the complex nature of structural poverty among black Americans, have thrown up their hands and moved on to helping other ethnic minorities.

The findings also strengthen the argument that many poor black women have few social roles other than those associated with motherhood. For women who use crack, even these roles are often difficult to accomplish. The social roles that many poor black women once looked to for self-esteem and identity shaping have nearly vanished from inner-city neighborhoods. In the past, black churches were community-based organizations. Communities were built around church membership. Regardless of socioeconomic status, women could assume high-status roles in churches, such as deaconesses, ushers, choir members, and "mothers" of the church (Hill Collins, 1991). Moreover, the results of the current study lead to better understanding of how the polarization of the American black population has affected the group that William Julius Wilson (1987) termed "the truly disadvantaged."

The findings express how role conflict is played out: Motherhood and crack use do not mix. The roles of each cannot exist in harmony with the other. As the results show, the crack-user role generally wins out over mothering. A few women decided to obtain drug treatment after they became pregnant, but the majority did not. Furthermore, most of the women who made the decision to seek drug treatment did not do so during all of their pregnancies. An important implication here is that in a weakened social structure, characterized by ambiguity of social ranks and responsibilities, a low-ranked role can overtake a higher-ranked role with little social pressure to stop the process. Put another way, in neighborhoods organized around crack sales, crack consumption, and sexual activities, fewer people occupy the stalwart roles that existed in these communities in the past. Motherhood was, at one time, ranked among the highest status a poor black women could achieve. In contrast, "crack user" is ranked among the lowest. Becoming a crack user has the ability to circumvent mothering for many poor black women, and this relates back to the weakened social structure and ambiguous social responsibilities that crack's introduction created in inner-city neighborhoods.

The findings of this study suggest that commitment to a role can be based on something other than rational choice. Commitment to maintain the crack-user role was strong for all of the women, and this commitment influenced the outcomes of their sex-for-crack pregnancies. The three women who chose to abort their sex-for-crack pregnancies made rational choices to do so in order to continue crack use. However, the majority of the women ignored their sex-for-crack pregnancies and continued to use crack until it was too late to safely have an abortion. They were committed to continuing crack use, but failed to make rational decisions concerning crack use and being pregnant. These women had their children by default as they continued to maintain the crack-user role. The anecdotal data suggest as well that pregnant users continue to exchange sex for crack. This phenomenon raises more questions than answers.

CRACK AND GENDER ROLES

Crack has shifted the balance of power between poor black men and women. The power women once held in their gender roles was lost when they began using crack cocaine and exchanging sex for crack. Crack has empowered some marginalized men within the crack-cocaine, underground economy. Poor black men, through crack, have obtained access to income denied to them by the larger society. More important, they have a powerful weapon to use in the battle between the sexes. These individuals, who had no economic opportunities before the drug's introduction, have surfaced as controlling agents in the crack culture. The evidence provided by the present study suggests that a gender role reversal has occurred.

Many poor black women, who have suffered rejection from the society at large, find their social position diminished within their own communities as a result of crack use. Thus, egalitarian gender roles being a characteristic of black families should be reevaluated as being a characteristic instead of middle-class blacks. The double standard for females in poor black communities is paradoxical indeed. As Kathy's experience demonstrates, male drug dealers have no problem selling drugs to women who are visibly pregnant. Male drug dealers will sell to pregnant women, and the anecdotal data suggest that these same men deride the women who use crack during pregnancy. To be sure, the pregnant women bear responsibility for exposing drugs to their unborn child; however, the men in these communities who sell drugs and participate in sex-for-crack exchanges should be held accountable for the results of their actions as well. The burden of nearly all of the repercussions of widespread crack addiction in inner cities rests on the shoulders of poor black women, whether they use crack or not. The women who use crack have the sole responsibility for children conceived by sex-for-crack exchange, and are held accountable for exposing their babies to crack before birth. The women's female, non–drug using relatives are frequently given the responsibility of raising these children. The men escape with minimal responsibility for any children they helped to produce.

Male drug dealers give little thought to the repercussions of their actions when they sell crack to pregnant women. The men in the crack world drift from one woman to the next, engaging in sexual intercourse with them, with no intent to establish commited relationships. Sexual behavior in this setting has evolved into a cash-and-carry business. People have become commodities for both sexes. For men, women are simply sexual toys; for women, men are providers of crack. Emotional attachment and love-based relationships as the basis of family formation is rare.

Poor black women are at a disadvantage due to the decline in male participation in families. Women are expected to be responsible for most family duties. Women who use crack are expected to do the same, in spite of their drug use. The results show that doing so is nearly impossible. The results also point out that the unbalanced gender roles prevalent in poor black families and crack's influence on these roles makes it difficult for families to remain stable.

The findings suggest that gender roles can change quickly as a result of sudden social and economic transitions. Thus, the results of the study lend support for the gender role theories expounded by E. Franklin Frazier (1939) and Charles Johnson (1934). These scholars emphasized the critical influences of slavery and the sharecropping system, which were the basis for gender role development among disadvantaged blacks.

The findings suggest as well that sex as a means of power and control is clearly evident in the sex-for-crack exchange system. The men who control crack can demand sex from any crack-using woman. The more crack a man has or has access to, the more powerful he is within the social structure. This kind of power, given to men who do not have legitimate jobs, is a heady experience. Poor black female crack users are often targeted for abuse. All of the women in the study stressed that men use crack to control women. Crack is an instrument of power that is used in the sexual contexts of users' lives. Men who possess crack can orchestrate who has sex with whom, determine which acts are performed, decide upon condom use, and determine the length of time the sexual acts continue. The French philosopher Michel Foucault's (1976) notion of the relationship between sex and power is supported in this analysis.

The "honeymoon phase" described in Chapter 6 suggests that the men who possess crack control women's statuses within the crack world. After a woman had exchanged sex for crack for a season, she became too familiar to the men. The men were constantly in search of different and younger women. Familiar women were derided and pushed out of the spotlight. The men often pay the familiar women less money or give less crack for sex acts. According to the qualitative data, the men also behave as though they were doing these women a favor. So, in addition to controlling crack distribution, the men control the women's relative ranking among other women. In this way, the men control who has access to crack, who has access to sexual partners, and decide upon the amount of cash or crack paid for sexual services.

As Foucault (1976) suggests, power is always met with resistance by those who are dominated by that power. The women in the study resisted the men's efforts to control their lives through partner selection, running crack houses, and developing tough street personas and conning skills. However, crack use limited the effectiveness of these strategies. This new social system created by crack has given men the masculine authority and status they could not achieve in the larger society. Recall that Moore (1969) stressed that poor black men experienced "masculinity without status." Masculinity without status refers to the phenomenon of being male without the means to fulfill traditional male gender roles, for example, a breadwinner job. In the crack world, the men appear to have status without norms. The men who have access to crack have status and authority without parameters or guidelines for exercising that authority.

The constraints of inner-city life offer few avenues to express that power. Sex is the only available option. The men exercise their authority by commanding women to have sex, and if the women challenge that authority, the men threaten to cut off the crack supply. Many men stretch the limits of their crack-endowed power, to see how far they can go and how far the women will go to continue access to crack. The women in the study shared tales of abuse, degradation, and humiliation they experienced and reported the abuse of women they knew. Foucault's (1976) treatise includes a discussion of Donatien Alphonse de Sade's (the Marquis de Sade) work. de Sade's notion of sex and sexuality is reminiscent of sex and sexuality among crack users. Foucault (1976) suggests that, "In Sade, sex is without any norms or intrinsic rule that might be formulated from its own nature; but it is subject to the unrestricted law of power which itself knows no other law but its own. . . . this exercise carries it to a point where it is no longer anything but a unique and naked sovereignty: an unlimited right of an all-powerful monstrosity" (p. 149). Similar to Sade's notion of sex, sex among crack users is more than the act itself. The act of sexual gratification is interwoven with the desire to harness power and authority over others. The marginalization of poor black men by the larger society created a power deficit. The frustrations and failures that poor black men experience trying to live up to mainstream norms for masculinity can be pushed aside if quantities of crack can be obtained.

This phenomenon makes clear why crack became so prevalent in inner cities. Access to crack can not only provide income and with it material possessions but also give powerless men instant status and unchallengeable authority. Access to crack makes the men in the ranks of the "poor marriage market" described by Wilson (1987) immediately appealing to women. With no experience in exercising authority, these men become intoxicated with the power access to crack gives and push this illegitimate power to the limit by forcing women to engage in degrading and humiliating sexual acts. Similar to de Sade, the men in the crack world use sex to dominate and achieve mastery over others. Most often, women are the targets of these power plays, and in the course of time assume "femininity without status" as gendered cultural power positions erode through crack-related humiliation and degradation. Thus the findings of this study and many others demonstrate that not all women benefited from the sexual emancipation that occurred during the 1960s and 1970s.

POLICY SUGGESTIONS

The behaviors of compulsive crack smokers have challenged conventional treatment applications, overwhelmed the social service industry, and shocked the nation with sensational stories of abuse and neglect, especially to children. The combination of risk-ridden sexual activity and crack use created the detrimental socializing mechanisms that characterize many inner-city poor communities. The rapid introduction of crack into these communities underscores their vulnerability and need for comprehensive and culturally competent strategies to address the myriad social pathologies plaguing poor black communities.

Lack of consideration for the cultural characteristics and social circumstances of addicted persons by treatment professionals is a major reason for program failure and substance abuse recidivism. Crack addiction and the sex-for-crack cocaine barter system are symptoms of underlying issues that have been ignored or minimally addressed by social policy. The findings of this research suggest policy formation in four areas: (1) drug treatment modification, (2) child welfare caseload evaluation, (3) inner-city public education policy, and (4) general social welfare policy.

Drug Treatment

First, the data suggest that drug treatment for poor black women of childbearing years should be modified substantially. Conventional treatment applications, such as twelve-step programs, have not been adequate to cope with their comprehensive problems. From a broad perspective, poor black women crack users suffer from societal exclusion with marginal educational and career opportunities. Life without these kinds of support systems makes recovery from drug abuse more difficult. More specifically, the black female crack user's experience is further complicated by the physical and social consequences of gender. Sex-for-crack pregnancies are evidence of these complications.

The findings support the need for drug treatment modification specifically designed for the unique characteristics of black women who exchange sex for crack. The findings demonstrate that the women have limited knowledge about their own bodies. Furthermore, the findings highlight the need for more comprehensive treatment that includes education seminars in human reproduction, pregnancy awareness training, and birth control methodology. Treatment components should include discussions of issues such as hormonal fluctuations and fertility. The findings also suggest that treatment facilities should include historical information on the black family and the importance of motherhood as a socializing mechanism and conduit for cultural stability. The importance of female gender roles in family life for the well-being of children should be stressed in treatment applications. This information may demonstrate that the violation of these traditions by crack use among poor black women and by sex-for-crack pregnancies affects the individuals involved as well as society. Furthermore, culture-based treatment components may help addicted women place their behavior in a larger context and stimulate thought processes that may lead to more responsible actions.

These discussions may help women understand the complex physical and social drives that influence them to become mothers. The treatment model may include suggestions for personal strategies to separate these drives from the context of sex-for-crack exchange. Education can empower the women and enable them to make more informed choices for their lives and the lives of their children. Furthermore, sex education learned in treatment facilities could be passed on to their daughters. General education and job training is needed as well. The data suggests that obtaining an education is problematic for a notable number of women. All of the women who participated in the ethnography were channeled into very-low-paying jobs that provided only subsistence wages. These findings make clear that in addition to drug treatment, women require opportunities to finish high school and to learn skills that can be marketed in the emerging technical economy.

Child Welfare

Second, the baseline data presented here may benefit child welfare agencies by providing empirical evidence that women are becoming pregnant by exchanging sex for crack and that children are produced in this way. This information should enhance the ability to evaluate their caseloads more efficiently. Children with this background may be more at risk for placement in foster care. Having the knowledge that a child was conceived in a sex-for-crack transaction may aid in the development of specific early intervention strategies geared to address their unique problems. Foster care placement may not be sufficient to meet these children's needs; additional services may be indicated, such as mental health therapy, self-esteem and conflict resolution training, and developmental therapy. These agencies may also use the data to assist in developing a profile of children at risk for abuse, neglect, or abandonment. Although no incidents of deliberate child abuse were discovered in this study, the potential for abuse existed. It is suspected that a five-year-old boy named "Terrell Peterson," who was murdered in 1998 in Atlanta, was a sex-for-crack–conceived child (Hansen, 1999; Visser, 2000).

The circumstances of his case, which were broadcast on television news shows and presented in newspapers, gave cause to think this was the case. Terrell's mother was reported to be a crack user. His mother had several older children who were placed in the custody of their paternal grandmother due to their mother's drug use. When Terrell was born, the child welfare agents sought to place him in the same home with his other siblings. However, the grandmother expressed reluctance to take Terrell. The grandmother clearly told the agents that Terrell was not fathered by her son, who was the father of the other children. Nevertheless, since the other children were well cared for they placed Terrell there as well. Without question, Terrell was not treated equally with the other children. The reports indicated that the child was tied up and deprived of food except for grits and oatmeal. He eventually died of an undeterminable blunt trauma, but the autopsy showed starvation played a role in his death as well.

Social welfare professionals assumed that the child would receive the same love and care as the other children. Obviously, there was more involved in this situation than they knew. If Terrell were truly conceived by sex for crack, the social welfare agents should never have placed the child in the home where he met his death. A more thorough probe into the life of the child's mother and the circumstances that predated his birth should have been undertaken. When the grandmother expressed reluctance to take the child, a red flag should have gone up and more information sought. For her, Terrell may have been a symbol of his mother's drug use and infidelity to her son. In cases such as these, the knowledge that a child was conceived by sex for crack could avoid hasty placement in an unsuitable home.

Public Education

The findings have strong implications for public education policy in poor urban schools. Children whose mothers use crack often have unstable life circumstances, whether living with their mothers or elsewhere. Children residing in the home of their crack-using mothers fare the worst. They are not guaranteed food, clean clothing, or, in some instances, a good night's rest. They may be left at home with no adult supervision at night or during the day. Some children (as described by April in Chapter 5) witness their mothers engaging in horrific acts in exchange for crack cocaine. A crack house may be the only home some children know, and, as the literature and the results of this study demonstrate, anything can happen in a crack house. Children who live under these conditions are at risk for not only exposure to sexual acts, violence, and degradation, but also for being targets of this kind of deviance simply by being there.

Children of crack-using mothers who live with relatives are also not guaranteed sufficient nurturing and stability. These children may be caught between loyalty to their mothers and loyalty to the custodial relative. Furthermore, the strategies the interviewed women used to maintain the highly valued role of motherhood may be disruptive in the children's life. Drifting in and out of children's lives in varying states of intoxication may confuse the children and set a dangerous precedent for the perception of "motherhood." Relatives who take responsibility for these children may be older, have limited income, and/or may have a number of children already in their care. In addition, these results suggest that family members willing to take care of the crack-using mother's children are becoming scarce, and they support recent claims of an overburdened foster care system.

Children in foster care do not always fare well either. This should always be the last resort when finding homes for children. However, the evidence from this analysis suggests that placement in multiple foster home situations predisposes children for negative life outcomes. Considering the number of simultaneous issues—the children of crack-using mothers, the concentration of extremely disadvantaged people, the emigration of stable middle- and working-class black families and the resulting decline in tax revenues to support schools—the inner-city public education systems' task of educating children is daunting. Schools in many inner cities all over the United States are finding it difficult to create an environment conducive to high-quality education. This is a complex dilemma embroiled in the historical, social, and economic issues described in Chapter 1. The loss of family-supporting jobs, the concentration of chronically poor people into one area, and the exodus of stable black families in the 1980s left many inner-city schools with a disproportionate number of children from families on public assistance.

As a result the increased proportion of poorer, less well-prepared children increased the demands on teachers to provide services outside of teaching. These services include parenting, disciplining, and teaching fundamental social skills, all of which should have been provided at home. This started the education system on a downward spiral and contributed to the current resegregation. Good teachers became disillusioned and began to seek employment elsewhere. As crack cocaine appeared on the landscape, additional stable families fled inner cities, and the schools became even more concentrated with children with disorganized home lives nearly devoid of adequate nurturing and preparation for a formal education environment.

Children with this kind of background would naturally have behavioral problems, for example, aggressive behavior, lack of self-control, attention-span deficits, along with difficulty concentrating, inability to remain seated for periods of time and follow classroom rules, talking while the teacher is teaching, and so on. When a teacher has many children in his or her class who have not be trained to control themselves, chaos ensues. That teacher may waste valuable teaching time by instead just trying to keep some semblance of order. The few children in the class who do not cause problems soon learn that the way to gain attention is to adopt deviant behaviors. A high turnover rate in teachers and administrators can be expected in situations such as these. This critical element must be considered in efforts to improve public schools in high-poverty census tracts. More money given to inner-city public schools is not the answer, but less money is not the answer either. Building social capital in poor communities may be part of the answer to this complex problem.

The concept of social capital has recently been applied to research on the relationship between poverty and poor health (Gold et al., 2002; Subramanian et al., 2003; Kennedy et al., 1998). Social capital is a concept developed by sociologist James Coleman (1988) and political scientist Robert Putman (2000). Social capital is defined as "those features of social organization—such as levels of interpersonal trust and norms of reciprocity and mutual aid—that facilitate collective action for mutual benefit" (Kawachi, 1999, p. 120) and exhibits strong social bonds, social cohesion, civic involvement, and mutual trust (Kawachi and Kennedy, 1997; Putman, 2000; Gold et al., 2002). These characteristics are diametrically opposed to characteristics of communities organized around crack consumption and distribution. As described in Chapter 3, the crack cocaine culture is selfish in nature, paranoid in its collective psychological element, and exploitative in human relationships. The crack stronghold in many poor inner-city communities strains any initiatives to shift focus away from self-gratification to cooperation for the benefit of educating young children. For the most part, social capital emigrated with the stable families and the breadwinner jobs that supported them. Rebuilding these communities is essential to saving the children.

Strategies to build social capital and change the landscape of inner-city public schools should begin by engaging communities and community leaders to identify their unique needs and concerns and to build partnerships with day care centers, church-based preschools, other preschools, and elementary schools. If no leaders can be identified, members of middle-class suburban communities should be enlisted to serve as temporary leaders until someone in the community can be identified and trained. These leaders should encourage the formation of community "watch-care" groups to ensure that all children in the neighborhood are receiving adequate care and nutrition, are supervised and protected, and are obtaining early home training.

Families affected by crack addiction should be targeted for educational interventions. Intensive mentoring programs for the women provide vital information regarding the importance of educating children at home in the early years (birth to age five). Crack-using women with young children should be required to have their children in preschools. Church-based preschools should consider providing free tuition for at-risk children. In addition, community "watch-care" groups should provide long-range support for the children as they enter middle and high schools.

These strategies are not new. During segregation, the stronger members of black communities "watched out" for children in struggling families for decades. Middle- and working-class blacks residing in comfortable suburbs should consider returning to the communities in which they grew up, or should seek out similar communities and volunteer to mentor children in need. Furthermore, middle- and working-class blacks should consider seeking funds for the development of private preschools and elementary schools in poor communities. These private schools should provide the same high-quality academic curricula and educational resources that many of the top-performing private schools employ, for example, A Beka, Saxon, Bob Jones, Alpha Omega, The Great Books Foundation, Wordly Wise, Writing Strands, Harcourt, University of Chicago, and Everyday Mathematics program, to name a few. Phonics-based reading skills and reading comprehension, problem-based mathematics, critical and logical thinking skills, science, and social studies should all be included in an academic grogram. Classroom size should be no more than twelve children per class in preschool through second grade, and no more than fifteen children per class in grades three through five. Selection for admission to a school should be on a first-come, first-served basis. No tuition should be required, however, parents should be required to partner with the school to ensure that the child attends class and keeps up with assignments. Parents should also provide appropriate corrective measures if discipline problems occur. If these criteria are not met, the children cannot attend the school. Establishing a school such as this in a poverty-stricken neighborhood, partnered with community "watch-care" group members and small community businesses, and with the help of large corporations or charitable institutions would greatly benefit many children. If children of crack-addicted mothers and other at-risk children are reached early and are supported through quality education, long-term community watch-care support, and family intervention, their lives can be charted on more productive courses.

Studying the workings of the black public education system during segregation can shed light on current inner-city education problems. It is not a coincidence that the decline in educational attainments of blacks in inner-city schools occurred after desegregation. Although segregated black schools did not have the same economic resources as their white counterparts, the great strength of these schools was the extraordinary teachers and administrators who worked there. School teaching and administration attracted the cream of the academic crop at that time because Jim Crow policy precluded the acquisition of other employment. Charles Murray's *Losing Ground: American Social Policy 1950-1980* (1984) describes a black school during segregation in Washington, DC, in which all employees had PhDs. Murray suggests that this situation was an anomaly, and indeed, this case may be extreme. However, a significant portion of black teachers in the past possessed graduate degrees. It was certainly true of the schools I attended. The principals of my junior high and high schools were both PhDs and many of my teachers either earned or were working on graduate degrees as well. These teachers left these schools after civil rights legislation became law to seek better-paying jobs, and the students lost many high-quality teachers.

The unfortunate consequence of desegregation was that these great teachers began leaving the school system for better paying jobs in the private sector, or they were sent to formerly white schools to "represent" the best of black teachers. Research on this subject may uncover successful teaching protocols of the past that can be utilized to improve current public education in urban areas.

General Social Welfare

Third, the findings of this study should direct policymakers to address two issues in general social policy: sex education policy and public policy toward poor blacks. First, appropriate sex education in public schools should be encouraged. Clearly, one of the most important discoveries in this research was that so many of the women did not receive adequate information about sex and reproduction before they reached sexual maturity. This controversial issue is still debated. This research makes clear that the absence of knowledge about sex can be a determinant of early sex and pregnancy. Other issues uncovered by the findings are the depth of marginalization of these women, the complexities of their lives, and how this impacts social policy toward poor blacks.

The welfare-to-work programs and the dramatic changes in welfare policy are tested by women such as those in the study. These women will be some of the hardest to place in self-sustaining jobs. Addiction to crack is only one obstacle. Lack of education, communication skills, and other marketable skills are other obstacles. Yet another obstacle to self-sufficiency is the lack of social support networks. The marginal work histories of the women in the study suggest a lack of exposure to the workweek cycle. These issues need to be addressed if the welfare system expects women with this background to obtain and keep jobs. It is important to remember that some of the women in the ethnography had never worked or worked only for very short periods of time. Society at large has unrealistic expectations of poor black female crack users. With all of the aforementioned negative circumstances, how can these women pull themselves up by the bootstraps? Only by years of retraining along with monetary and social support from non–drug users.

The question is this: Is society willing to invest the time, effort, and money into people they consider undesirable? Conservative politicians' quests to dismantle welfare has been motivated by the image of undeserving, drug-using welfare mothers. These are the women who require the most resources to place them in the workforce. Cutting off their public assistance makes the problem even larger. Where do they turn? Politicians who support completely cutting the women off from all sources of aid must be prepared for increased crime, more homelessness, and worsening social conditions in inner cities.

I am not against a revamping of welfare. However, much money will have to be spent to prepare the poorest of the poor for social roles that they have never occupied before. This issue is reminiscent of the controversial historic debate between Booker T. Washington and W. E. B. Du Bois concerning the education of newly freed slaves in the latter part of the nineteenth century.

Booker T. Washington stressed industrial and technical education for blacks after emancipation. His goal was to groom blacks to occupy service-sector jobs and for ownership of land for farming. W. E. B. Du Bois stressed that higher learning was the path to full citizenship for blacks. As with other issues concerning blacks in the United States, such as those discussed in Chapter 2, the dichotomy of philosophies failed to demonstrate to scholars that more than one solution to a problem may exist. Today we are faced with a dilemma similar to that faced in the post-emancipation years. Thousands of blacks who are peripheral to the economy require merger into the system. No single solution will be appropriate for all. Both Washington's and Du Bois' ideas should be revisited and considered for channeling the thousands, perhaps millions, of poor black people currently involved in the crack social organization structure into mainstream social and economic roles. Their polemic should suggest to policymakers today that a single social policy is not adequate to address the diversity extant within the American black population. Furthermore, the economic shifts and bifurcation of the black population closed the windows of opportunity for lower classes to achieve upward mobility. Unless initiatives are taken to improve the eroded inner-city education systems and to increase underclass exposure to middle-class role models, the middle class will most likely remain static and then decline due to the tendency toward smaller families. The underclass will continue to grow, given their tendency to have larger families.

Public policy toward blacks has turned cold in recent years. The wax and wane of public policy toward American blacks is reminiscent of a very slow, upward escalator moving toward the promised land of self-sufficiency. This escalator is powered by opportunity structures such as education and access to family-supporting jobs, and has been turned off and on since reconstruction. People at the top are generally closely associated with the mainstream and have access to opportunities for making progress. As they disembark, they are replaced by others, slowly making their way to the top. In the 1980s and

1990s, dramatic changes in the public policy toward blacks shifted and the escalator came to a stop. Only those closest to the top with strong connections to the power source can now climb to the top and disembark, leaving a crowd of people at the bottom, struggling to get on a malfunctioning conveyer.

CONCLUSIONS

Social and economic forces that resulted in masses of unemployed black males and established the single-parent, female-headed household as the dominant family pattern created the optimum conditions for a crack cocaine stronghold in inner cities. The combined and often multiplicative effects of race, class, and gender marginalization experienced by poor black women increased their vulnerability to exchanging sex for crack. Moreover, the urgency of crack addiction interferes with self-protection strategies, such as condom use. Pregnancies conceived by sex-for-crack exchange occurred in more than half of the women in the study who engaged in this behavior. Despite the circumstances that produced the pregnancies, the importance of motherhood to the self-concept of the women, the minimal importance of biological fatherhood, and religious beliefs influenced most of the women to carry the babies to term. In sharp contrast, increased crack consumption prevented them from taking responsibility for the well-being of the child during gestation.

The women in the study were themselves neglected as children. Most did not receive adequate knowledge about their sexuality in time enough to empower and protect themselves against unplanned pregnancies. Information about sex and reproduction was avoided by their caregivers. Perhaps this was done to protect them against the highly sexual image of black women held by the larger society and within the inner-city communities. This attempt at protection had the opposite effect: it rendered the women vulnerable by not informing them of what to expect from their changing bodies and from the men in their lives. The nonconfrontational approach to sexuality was carried over into avoidance behavior when coping with the repercussions of sexuality in the crack world.

Prostitution and sex for crack differ in fundamental ways. Prostitutes generally protect themselves from pregnancies with clients. Sex for crack is associated with desperation and a lack of concern for the possibility of conceptions. This behavior has strong social implications. Children born outside of a socially accepted sexual union are generally stigmatized. Moreover, children born under sex-for-crack circumstances generally are few in number in most societies. Sex-for-crack–conceived children may experience social repercussions that are yet unknown. The lives they live in unstable families further complicate their troubled beginnings. This study clearly points out that these families require help, not only from the federal government, but also from private citizens, churches, corporations, small businesses, blacks, whites, and everyone in the United States who is currently living the American dream. Society has a responsibility to address this social problem that the American political economy helped to create.

Chapter 10

Method Notes

OVERVIEW

Social epidemiological procedures were used to locate poor black female crack users, to distinguish women who exchanged sex for crack on a regular basis, and to identify those who became pregnant this way. The outcomes of sex-for-crack pregnancies were ascertained as well. Ethnographic interviews were conducted with the women who became pregnant to obtain in-depth information and to identify cultural and other influences on sex-for-crack pregnancy outcomes. Thus, two interview instruments were developed and used for two distinct interviews. One instrument, a short, coded screening device, was used to interview a larger screening sample of women. This instrument was used to determine subject eligibility, identify a theoretical sample, and collect fundamental and demographic data from every woman contacted. The second instrument, a much longer, semistructured interview guide, was used with the theoretical sample of women who became pregnant by exchanging sex for crack cocaine. This instrument was used to capture and probe the details of sex-for-crack pregnancies as they impact the women's lives. In addition, a focus group was held with eight poor black female crack users in a drug treatment setting. The focus group was used in an exploratory capacity to develop the two aforementioned instruments and for orientation to current street terminology.

BACKGROUND AND PROJECT SEQUENCE

A research design was chosen that could accommodate multiple methodologies. Moreover, an approach was required to assess the prevalence and outcomes of sex-for-crack pregnancies and to provide an accurate interpretation of influences on these phenomena from the women's perspectives, apart from social commentary and sensationalism. The qualitative research tradition allows the research craftsperson to select from a broad range of data collection and analysis methods, descriptive devices, and interpretive paradigms. In addition, the qualitative design does not preclude the use of quantitative data in tandem with textual data (Denzin and Lincoln, 1998). Two metaphors of qualitative research influenced the choices made for this project. First, Valerie Janesick's model of qualitative research as dance provided the basis for the organization of the project, the development of the role of the researcher, and was central to the conception of data triangulation (Janesick, 1998). For Janesick, the steps in the process of qualitative research are similar to the steps a choreographer uses when developing and staging a dance.

In the *warm-up* phase, I prepared to enter the field by contacting several key informants I met in the context of another project on women and drug use, held meetings with them, and obtained letters of commitment from them indicating that they would assist in recruiting research respondents. The warm-up phase was rather lengthy. The initial contacts were made in the summer of 1997 as I prepared a National Institutes of Health National Institute on Drug Abuse grant application to seek support for the project. I received funding and began the research process in April of 1998.

At that time, I met with the key informants again and arranged a temporary research space at two facilities: an inpatient treatment facility and a grassroots, drop-in, self-help center. Both facilities are located in known areas of drug sales and consumption. During this phase the interview instruments were developed. The data collection or *performance* phase began in May of 1998 and continued until September of 1998. I established rapport with potential research subjects by speaking before several groups of women in both locations. I shared details of my background and research with the women and the professionals working there, and stressed their importance in the process. By doing so, I created a temporary role for myself in the two settings that allowed me to conduct interviews with relative simplicity. The first screening interviews and the focus group were conducted. The interview instruments were refined. Most of the screening and in-depth interviews were conducted during this phase. When my data collection was completed, in the *cool-down* phase, I produced and submitted final reports of my activities in each setting. During the cool-down period, a few more women were screened and interviewed. The gradual process of leaving the field began in October of 1998 and lasted until January of 1999 when the final reports were submitted.

Valerie Janesick also stresses the importance of including multiple data sources and multiple methods for the study of a single phenomenon. Triangulation, then, can be built into a research process at the outset (Janesick, 1998). The present study incorporated three data sources: screening interviews, in-depth interviews, and a focus group, as well as two methodologies: a variation of social epidemiology and an ethnography. The combination of raw materials adds depth to the understanding of the phenomenon of sex-for-crack exchange among poor black women.

The other metaphor of qualitative research that I drew upon is qualitative research as bricolage. Drawing from French anthropologist Claude Levi-Straus, Denzin and Lincoln (1998) convey that bricolage is "a pieced together, close-knit set of practices that provide solutions to a problem in a concrete situation" (Denzin and Lincoln, 1998, p. 3). This model guided my data collection, analysis, and interpretation choices, and defined the parameters of the end product. With this framework in mind, the end product should resemble an organized and integrated collage or patchwork quilt of information and processes that provide a clear and meaningful picture of sex-for-crack exchange as a mechanism that produces pregnancies in the specified sample of women. Furthermore, this design principle allowed me as "bricoleur" to acknowledge my background, strengths and weaknesses, and biases along with those of the research participants, which together shaped the research and writing processes. In addition, the bricoleur understands that the results of the research do not exist in a vacuum and will ultimately have public policy implications (Denzin and Lincoln, 1998).

PROJECT-PARTICIPANT PROFILE

A project-participant profile was developed to ensure that only women who were representative of the social, economic, and cultural concerns of this project described in Chapter 1 were selected for the screening sample and the theoretical sample. Subject eligibility was verified verbally by key informants before selection for participation in the screening sample and was based on the following criteria:

1. *Race:* Subjects must be black and born in the United States.
2. *Age:* Subjects must currently be adults of childbearing age or adults who were of childbearing age in 1985. The range of ages is anticipated to be eighteen to fifty. Many researchers cite 1985 as the year that crack-cocaine addiction in inner-city poverty areas reached epidemic proportions and became visible to the rest of the country (Inciardi et al., 1993; Williams, 1989). A thirty-seven-year-old woman addicted to crack in 1985 would have been approaching her fiftieth birthday the year the study was conducted. This was the rationale behind the extended range of ages. A wide range of subject ages allowed comparison of experiences between women who began crack use at the beginning of the epidemic and those who started after the culture had become entrenched within the inner-city social structure.
3. *Drug-use pattern:* Subjects must be smokers of crack cocaine (as opposed to those who snort or inject cocaine) and use the drug at least three times per week.
4. *Habit support:* Subjects must support their drug habit by sex-for-crack cocaine exchange. Support their drug habit by sex for crack grants the women the title of "addict" by researchers in the substance abuse field (Bourgois, 1989; Inciardi, 1989; Inciardi et al., 1993; Ratner, 1993). Exchanging sex for crack is considered a symptom of addiction, regardless of the frequency of crack consumption. Exchanging sex for crack generally occurs after compulsive use becomes addiction and after other resources to purchase the drug have been exhausted (Ratner, 1993). By definition, this criteria is the project marker for addiction.
5. *Treatment status:* Subjects must be currently addicted to crack and have been in drug treatment for six months or less at the time of contact. Women in treatment must have used crack cocaine at least three times per week and exchanged sex for crack to support the drug habit during their addiction.
6. *Socioeconomic status:* Subjects must be from poverty-stricken, inner-city areas previously described and earn less than $10,000 per year at a legitimate job.

SCREENING AND SAMPLING PROCESSES

Research participants were drawn with purposive- and snowball-sampling procedures. In purposive sampling, selection of subjects was based on specific criteria relevant to the research purposes. The criteria for selection are listed in the previous section. Snowball sampling is a methodology that initiates referral chains of subjects, starting with one subject. Two phases, informal and formal screening processes, were used to locate poor black female crack users who met the aforementioned criteria. Key informants were used to informally identify and/or recruit the crack users. Informal screening at homeless shelters, the inpatient treatment center, and the storefront self-help center were also conducted. Informal screening consisted of casually talking with women and asking about drug use and related experiences. Likely candidates were interviewed with the formal screening device. Women were not told that I was interested in finding women who became pregnant by exchanging sex for crack; they were told that I was interested in the experiences of women who exchange sex for crack. Details about the in-depth interview and compensation for it were not disclosed during the screening process. These measures were taken to ensure more honest answers to the questions. After the screening interview, women were asked for referrals of other women who exchanged sex for crack to start the snowball chain. More than sixty poor black women were informally screened. Fifty-two crack users were identified and formally screened to confirm project eligibility. Forty-six women met all project criteria.

Short Screening Instrument Description

All of the questions on the formal screening instrument were the closed-ended coded type. Items included such demographic information as age and education, drug-use frequency and last crack use, sex-for-crack frequency, HIV testing and status, condom and other birth control use, drug treatment involvement, homelessness status, and sexually transmitted disease frequency. They were also asked such defining questions as: Have you ever become pregnant by exchanging sex for crack? How many times has this happened? and What was/were the pregnancy outcomes? The pregnancy outcomes were coded as follows: (1) abortion, (2) miscarriage, (3) live birth, (4) still birth, (5) tubal pregnancy, and (6) pregnant now.

This instrument was constructed so that the pregnancy outcomes and basic information on each woman could be obtained at first contact. This way, if the women who were eligible to be included in the theoretical sample were lost or did not participate in the longer interview, the outcomes of their sex-for-crack pregnancies could still be documented. The short screening interview was completed in two to three minutes. Women were not compensated for participation in the short interview. The short screening instrument was used to identify women who exchange sex for crack, to identify women who became pregnant by sex-for-crack exchange, to ascertain the outcomes of the pregnancies, and to ensure that background data were collected from every woman contacted.

ETHNOGRAPHY

The ethnographic component of the research was based on two sources of data: a focus group and in-depth interviews. First, a focus group was held with eight women who met the project requirements. The focus group served a dual purpose. The session was conducted early in the project and informed the development of the in-depth interview instrument and refinement of the screening instrument. This data source served as a foundation for building this part of the research and added significantly to the textual database. Second, the primary source of ethnographic data was the product of the in-depth interviews. These data were comprehensive and gave rich descriptions of the behaviors associated with exchanging sex for crack cocaine.

Theoretical Sample

Theoretical sampling is a process of selecting subjects according to their relevance to the research questions. The screening process identified these individuals. After the administration of the formal screening questionnaire, women who reported that they had become pregnant by sex-for-crack exchange were asked to participate in a longer, in-depth interview. Twenty-three women were eligible for the theoretical sample. Interviews were conducted with nineteen of the twenty-three women who became pregnant by sex-for-crack exchange. Two women were lost in the crack street scene before interviews could be conducted. Some in-depth information was gathered from one of the women lost to follow up. She participated in the focus group held during the formative phase of the research. Two women declined to be interviewed.

The In-Depth Interview Instrument

A semistructured instrument was designed to capture coded demographic data and ethnographic descriptions of behaviors, relationships, and cultural patterns within the crack world. This instrument included questions concerning drug use during pregnancy, family structure, sexual risk taking, condom and other birth control use, and prostitution history, as well as a detailed analysis of each sex-for-crack pregnancy, pregnancy outcomes, and reasons for outcomes. The women were asked to answer the following questions concerning each sex-for-crack pregnancy: What role did the status of the father (drug user, unknown, etc.) have in the decision concerning the pregnancy? What role did religious beliefs have in the decision-making process? Did drug use influence the decision, and if so, why? The subject was also asked to identify other key issues that influenced the decision to carry a baby to term or have an abortion.

The women were asked a series of questions related to risk cognition while engaging in sex for crack. Simply put, they were asked: While engaging in unprotected sex for crack, do you ever think about getting pregnant or contracting sexually transmitted disease, including HIV? Why or why not? Questions probing knowledge about sex and reproduction were included as well. The women were also asked to estimate how many times per week they engaged in unprotected sex for crack.

Open-ended questions addressed the emotional state of the women who experienced the loss of children through legal or other intervention, miscarriages, or abortion. These questions were designed to establish a link between emotional trauma of these losses and additional pregnancies. Specifically, the women were asked: After losing a child, did you become pregnant again? How soon did you become pregnant again? Why do you think you became pregnant again? Do you think losing a child influenced you to become pregnant? Why?

If the sex-for-crack pregnancy resulted in the birth of a child, the details of each child's life circumstances were probed (for example, who had custody?). Questions about the child's quality of life were also asked such as: Does the child have emotional or physical disabilities? If yes, the mother was asked to detail the difficulties. How well the child performed in school was also asked. Mothers were asked if they thought their sex-for-crack children were treated differently than those not conceived by sex for crack and to explan their thoughts on the issue. They were also asked to identify who treated the child differently by first name only.

The mothers were asked to describe their relationships with the children, their emotional attachment to them, and to detail their lives together. The women were also asked questions about the meaning of motherhood, the changes in mothering brought about by crack use, and were asked to estimate the amount of time, in hours per day, they spent mothering their children. They were also asked to describe how they managed to be a good mother while using crack.

Open-ended questions probed the potential for abuse, abandonment, and neglect of sex-for-crack children, for example: Has the child ever been abused? If the answer was yes, a series of coded and open-ended questions were asked concerning the type of abuse, the abuser, and the circumstances surrounding the occurrences. The mother was also asked how well the child got along with others and why.

Additional Questions

Other questions addressing background issues, such as the meaning of fatherhood, the importance of a two-parent family structure as opposed to a single-parent family structure, the roles in the crack world, the roles in mainstream life, life before crack, relationships with men, and self-esteem were also included on this comprehensive interview guide. A variant of the Rosenberg self-esteem scale was administered as well (Rosenberg, 1965).

The first drafts of the screening device and the in-depth instrument were pretested and updated with the focus group data. The instruments were further tested with the first five subjects who were recruited from the street. Additional revisions were made upon the discovery of important issues.

In-Depth Interview Process

Each interview began with a thorough briefing on the nature of the research. The importance of the subject's contribution to the study was emphasized. Informed consent was administered to each subject and signed before starting the interview. The issues of subject anonymity and confidentiality were explained in detail. The interviews were recorded on audio tape and were erased after transcribing.

Data Management

Each recorded interview was transcribed as soon as possible for data accuracy and entered into a computer database file. Hard copies of each interview transcription were printed and filed numerically in a folder with the interview guide used for that interview. These measures reduced the likelihood of lost data. The signed consent forms were filed separately. All program documents and data were secured in a locked filing cabinet.

HUMAN SUBJECTS' CONCERNS

Approval from the Institutional Review Board at Georgia State University was obtained March 12, 1998, for the first year and January 1999 for the second year of the project. All subjects who agreed to participate in the study were not harmed physically or emotionally. The researcher worked in conjunction with experienced street recruiters to ensure that each individual was treated with respect and diplomacy during the recruiting and interview process. Prior to any research activities, each project participant was thoroughly briefed on the nature of the study and administered informed consent. The importance of the research topic and the subject's role in the process was explained. This consent form also detailed the issues of confidentiality and anonymity. The research participant's right to refuse to answer any question or terminate the interview at any time was explained. Data management techniques that were used ensured that the interview transcripts did not contain subject-identifying markers, and were filed separately from signed consent forms. Subjects were informed that if active child abuse was discovered during the interview, it would be reported to the proper authorities.

DATA ANALYSIS

Qualitative Data

All textual material was analyzed with constant comparative analysis, a component of the grounded theory method for qualitative data analysis (Strauss and Glaser, 1967; Strauss and Corbin, 1990). The constant comparative analysis was a rigorous process that allowed the researcher to discover themes and patterns in qualitative data during the entire process of the research. The text of the qualitative interviews and of the focus group transcript were read and entered into the database. Concepts were coded and given tentative labels during the open phase of the coding process. Open coding is a process of comparing concepts found in text for classification as examples of behaviors or relationships. As similarities in experience, patterns, and emergent themes appeared, categories of phenomena were labeled and entered into a code list. The categories consisted of groupings of phenomena that represent a more abstract quality. Core or central categories were the roots that anchored other categories. Text excerpts were categorized as examples of or related to the core categories, and were designated by the appropriate code. Theoretical saturation was reached when in-depth interview number 17 was completed, after which no new categories were ascertained. A model of sex-for-crack exchange behavior and pregnancies was developed by determining which patterns occurred most often and by linking behaviors to social contexts.

Quantitative Data

The quantitative data produced with the screening device, along with the coded questions and measurement scales from the in-depth instrument, were entered into two separate computer databases and analyzed with the Statistical Package for Social Sciences (SPSS). Descriptive statistics were produced for all of the variables in these databases. A demographic profile of poor black women who exchange sex for crack was developed. Characteristics of those who have become pregnant by exchange were determined. Profiles of those who have not become pregnant were produced as well. Outcomes of sex-for-crack pregnancies were ascertained. Variables such as frequency of drug use and sex-for-crack frequency were produced. A number of statistical procedures were executed, for example, cross tabs and chi square, t-tests, and several others, to discover relationships among the variables. The small sample size precluded the meaningful interpretation of most of these analyses.

Special Concerns

The personal nature of the research required a subtle approach, undergirded by an atmosphere of encouragement and diplomacy. I approached each potential participant in a straightforward but sensitive manner. I indicated that I was interested in talking to black women who use crack. At first, the women viewed me with skepticism. Many of the female crack users were so ashamed of their lives that they avoided eye contact. I tried to establish eye contact first. Then, I gave explanations for my interest in them. I am truly committed to finding help for these women through research, and I tried to share that with them. I also explained that their stories were important. I stressed the importance of telling the truth so that the true experience of black female crack users could be known. Furthermore, I stressed the importance of their lives also.

End Note

Although many studies have been conducted among poor black female crack users, I sought to do a number of things differently with this research. First, I wanted to frame their experiences with social, economic, and historical contexts to demonstrate that the behaviors described here did not just appear. The behaviors and attitudes in the crack world are anchored in the long historic expression of sex, race, and class marginalization. Second, I wanted to stress the complexity and severity of these women's problems with everyday life to demonstrate how difficult it is for most of them to simply get through a day. From the beginning of their lives, the severest structural limitations held dreams for jobs, relationships, and families to a very low standard. Third, the crack world exists in parallel to mainstream American culture. I wanted to cut across the divide and bring the stories of these women to readers who may otherwise never know such stories. I hope that the words in this book will spark a national movement to help these women and their children.

Glossary

cook it up: The process of mixing cocaine powder with baking soda, water, and sometimes other chemicals, and applying heat to produce a precipitate: crack.

crack house: A house, apartment, shed, or any abandoned shelter that has been commandeered purposefully by drug dealers or serendipitously by attrition for the sale of, consumption of, or sex in exchange for crack cocaine.

date: A trick; a person who will pay for sex with a crack prostitute.

DFACS: The Department of Family and Children Services; the state agency that acts to protect children. They also are responsible for the administration of public aid.

dope trap: A place where dope is sold. Usually an alley, abandoned apartment, or shed. Most of the time dope traps are not conducive for sexual activities.

eight ball: An eight ball is a large crack rock equivalent to an eighth of an ounce of cocaine. This is one of the largest quantities dispensed on the street.

geek: As a noun: the street descriptive term for one who uses crack and exhibits the paranoid behavior associated with crack use. As a verb: to use crack.

geek and freak: The street term for the crack use and prostitution binging cycle; using crack, followed by turning tricks, followed by using more crack, followed by more tricks, and so on.

geeked: High on crack, as in *geeked up*.

hit: As a noun: an inhale of crack smoke; a draw or two on the beverage can, pipe, or straight shooter on which the drug is burned. As a verb: to inhale the crack smoke.

house hit: The courtesy draw of smoke provided by a patron entering a crack house.

nicks: A five dollar quantity of crack. Other values of crack include dimes (ten dollars' worth) and twenties (twenty dollars' worth).

sack: A plastic bag containing a small amount of crack.

smoke house: A house or apartment in which the residents allow people who purchase crack elsewhere to use it for consuming crack. This is another economic opportunity provided by the crack fiscal system.

smoke out: A crack party.

trick: A prostitution client.

References

Anderson, Elijah. 1978. *A Place on the Corner*. Chicago: University of Chicago Press.

Anderson, Elijah. 1990. *Streetwise: Race, Class, and Change in an Urban Community*. Chicago: University of Chicago Press.

Bachman, Jerald, Wallace, John, O'Malley, Patrick, Johnston, Lloyd, Kurth, Candace, and Neighbors, Harold. 1991. "Racial/Ethnic Differences in Smoking, Drinking and Illicit Drug Use Among American High School Seniors, 1976-1989." *American Journal of Public Health* 81(3): 372-377.

Bass, Lessie and Jackson, Mary S. 1997. "A Study of Drug Abusing African American Pregnant Women." *Journal of Drug Issues* 27(3): 659-671.

Bateman, David A., Ng, Stephen K. C., Hansen, Catherine A., and Heagarty, Margaret C. 1993. "The Effects of Intrauterine Cocaine Exposure in Newborns." *American Journal of Public Health* 83(2): 190-193.

Beaty-Muller, Rachel and Boyle, Joyceen S. 1996. "You Don't Ask for Trouble: Women Who Do Sex and Drugs." *Family Community Health* 19(3): 35-48.

Becker, Howard. 1953. *Outsiders: Studies in the Sociology of Deviance*. New York: The Free Press.

Bernard, Jessie. 1966. *Marriage and Family Among Negroes*. New Jersey: Prentice-Hall.

Billingsley, Andrew. 1968. *Black Families in White America*. Englewood Cliffs, New Jersey: Prentice-Hall.

Billingsley, Andrew. 1992. *Climbing Jacob's Ladder*. New York: Simon & Schuster.

Blackwell, James E. 1975. *The Black Family Community Diversity and Unity*. New York: Dodd, Mead and Company.

Blanton, Marsha, Anthony, James, and Schuster, Charles. 1993. "Probing the Meaning of Racial/Ethnic Group Comparisons in Crack Cocaine Smoking." *Journal of the American Medical Association* 269(8): 993-997.

Booth, Robert E., Watters, John, and Chitwood, Dale. 1993. "HIV Risk Related Sex Behaviors Among Injection Drug Users, Crack Smokers, and Injection Drug Users Who Smoke Crack." *American Journal of Public Health* 83(8): 1144-1148.

Bourgois, Phillipe. 1989. "In Search of Horatio Alger: Culture and Ideology in the Crack Economy." *Contemporary Drug Problems*. Winter: 619-649.

Bourgois, Phillipe. 1996. "In Search of Masculinity: Violence, Respect and Sexuality among Puerto Rican Crack Dealers in East Harlem." *British Journal of Criminology* 36(3): 412-416.

Bowman, Phillip. 1993. "The Impact of Economic Marginality among African American Husbands and Fathers." In Harriette Pipes McAdoo (Ed.), *Family Ethnicity* (pp. 120-137). Newbury Park, CA: Sage Publications.

Burns, William J. and Burns, Kayreen A. 1988. "Parenting Dysfunction in Chemically Dependent Women." In Ira J. Chasnoff (Ed.), *Drugs, Alcohol, Pregnancy and Parenting* (pp. 159-169). Boston: Kluwer Academic Publishers.

Centers for Disease Control and Prevention. 2005. HIV and AIDS Surveillance Report: Cases of HIV Infections and AIDS in the United States, 2003. Volume 15. March 14. Atlanta, GA: Author.

Chasnoff, I. J., Griffith, D. R., MacGregor, D. O., Dirkes, K., and Burns, K. A. 1989. "Temporal Patterns of Cocaine Use in Pregnancy." *Journal of the American Medical Association* 261: 1741-1744.

Coleman, James. 1988. "Social Capital in the Creation of Human Capital." *American Journal of Sociology* 94(Suppl.): S95-S120.

Coontz, Stephanie. 1992. *The Way We Never Were: American Families and the Nostalgia Trap.* New York: Basic Books.

Cross, J. C., Johnson, B. D., Davis, W. Rees, and Liberty, H. J. 2001. "Supporting the Habit: Income Generation Activities of Frequent Crack Users Compared with Frequent Users of Other Hard Drugs." *Drug and Alcohol Dependence* 64: 191-201.

Darity, William and Myers, Samuel. 1992. "Sex Ratios, Marriage-ability and the Marginalization of African American Men." *The Challenge* 3(1): 5-13.

Davis, Angela. 1995. "Reflections on the Black Women's Role in the Community of Slaves." In Beverly Guy-Sheftall (Ed.), *Words of Fire: An Anthology of African-American Feminist Thought* (pp. 200-219). New York: The New Press.

Dembo, Richard. 1993. "Crack Cocaine Dealing by Adolescents in Two Public Housing Projects: A Pilot Study." *Human Organization* 52(1): 89-96.

Denzin, Norman and Lincoln, Yvonna. 1998. "Introduction: Entering the Field of Qualitative Research." In Norman Denzin and Yvonna Lincoln (Eds.), *Strategies of Qualitative Inquiry* (pp. 1-34). Thousand Oaks, CA: Sage Publications.

Devine, Joel A. and Wright, James D. 1993. *The Greatest of Evils: Urban Poverty and the American Underclass.* New York: Aldine De Gruyter.

Dill, Bonnie Thorton. 1990. "The Dialectics of Black Womanhood." In Micheline Malson, Elisabeth Mudimbe-Boyi, Jean O'Barr, and Mary Wyer (Eds.), *Black Women in America: Social Science Perspectives* (pp. 65-77). Chicago: University of Chicago Press.

Dunlap, Eloise and Johnson, Bruce. 1992. "The Setting for the Crack Era: Macro Forces, Micro Consequences: 1960-1992." *Journal of Psychoactive Drugs* 24(4): 307-321.

Duster, Troy. 1997. "Pattern, Purpose and Race in the Drug War." In Craig Reinarman and Harry Levine (Eds.), *Crack in America: Demon Drugs and Social Justice* (pp. 260-287). Berkeley: University of California Press.

Elshtain, Jean Bethke. 1990. "Pregnancy Police." *The Progressive* 54(12): 26-28.

Elwood, W. N., Williams, M. L., Bell, D. C., and Richard, A. J. 1997. "Powerlessness and HIV Prevention Among People Who Trade Sex for Drugs ('Strawberries')." *AIDS Care* 9(3): 273-284.

Feagin, Joe and Feagin, Clairece. 1993. *Racial and Ethnic Relations.* Englewood Cliffs, NJ: Prentice-Hall.

Forney, Mary Ann, Inciardi, James, and Lockwood, Dorothy. 1992. "Exchanging Sex for Crack Cocaine: A Comparison of Women from Rural and Urban Communities." *Journal of Community Health* 17(2): 73-85.

Foucault, Michel. (1976) *The History of Sexuality: An Introduction,* Volume 1. New York: Vantage Books.

Franklin, John Hope. 1969. *From Slavery to Freedom, A History of Negro Americans.* New York: Vintage Books.

Frazier, E. Franklin. 1939. *The Negro Family in the United States.* Chicago: University of Chicago Press.

Frazier, E. Franklin. 1957. *The Black Bourgeoisie.* New York: The Free Press.

Freeman, Edith M. 1994. "African American Women and the Concept of Cultural Competence." *Journal of Multicultural Social Work* 3(4): 61-76.

Fullilove, Mindy Thompson, Lown, E. Anne, and Fullilove, Robert. 1992. "Crack Ho's and Skeezers: Traumatic Experiences of Women Crack Users." *The Journal of Sex Research* 29(2): 275-287.

Gelb, Adam. 1990. "Bankhead Courts, A Comeback." *Atlanta Journal-Constitution.* December 30: B-01.

Geter, Robert S. 1994. "Drug User Settings: A Crack House Typology." *The International Journal of the Addictions* 29(8): 1015-1027.

Giddings, Paula. 1984. *When and Where I Enter.* New York: William Morrow and Company.

Gilmore, Mary R. 1990. "Racial Differences in Acceptability and Availability of Drugs and Early Initiation of Substance Use." *American Journal of Drug and Alcohol Abuse* 16(3/4): 185-206.

Gold, Rachel, Kennedy, Bruce, Connell, Fred, and Kawachi, Ichiro. 2002. "Teen Births, Income Inequality, and Social Capital: Developing an Understanding of the Causal Pathway." *Health and Place* 8: 77-83.

Goldstein, Paul. 1979. *Prostitution and Drugs.* Lexington, MA: Lexington Books.

Goldstein, Paul J., Ouellet, Lawrence J., and Fendrich, Michael. 1992. "From Bag Brides to Skeezers: A Historical Perspective on Sex-for-Drugs Behavior." *Journal of Psychoactive Drugs* 24(4): 349-361.

Green, Nanny L. 1994. "Low Birth Weight and Infant Mortality in the African American Family: The Impact of Racism and Self Esteem." In Robert Staples (Ed.), *The Black Family* (pp. 187-194). Belmont, CA: Wadsworth Publishing Company.

Guttman, Herbert. 1976. *The Black Family in Slavery and Freedom, 1750-1925.* New York: Pantheon.

Hannerz, Ulf. 1969. *Soulside: Inquiries into Ghetto Culture and Community.* New York: Columbia University Press.

Hansen, Jane. 1998a. "Growing Up with Crack Series Part 1: A Forsaken Generation." *Atlanta Journal-Constitution.* September 27: A1, A16, A17.

Hansen, Jane. 1998b. "Growing Up with Crack Series Part 2: Hitting the Rock in Jurassic Park." *Atlanta Journal-Constitution.* September 28: A1.

Hansen, Jane. 1998c. "Growing Up with Crack Series Part 3: When They Can't Go Home." *Atlanta Journal-Constitution.* September 29: A1, A10, A11.

Hansen, Jane. 1998d. "Growing Up with Crack Series Part 4: Family First System Puts Children Last." *Atlanta Journal-Constitution.* September 30: A1.

Hansen, Jane. 1998e. "Growing Up with Crack Series Part 5: Parents Again." *Atlanta Journal-Constitution.* October 1: A1.

Hansen, Jane. 1999. "Did 5-Year-Old Terrell Have to Die?" *Atlanta Journal-Constitution.* October 17. Available online at: http://www.gahsc.org/terrell/terrell.html.

Hassan, An el-Fawal and Wood, Ronald. 1995. "Airway Smooth Muscle Relaxant Effects of the Cocaine Pyrolysis Product, Methylecgonidine." *Journal of Pharmacology and Experimental Therapeutics* 272(3): 991-996.

Hatchett, Shirley J. and Jackson, James S. 1993. "African American Extended Kin Systems." In Harriette Pipes McAdoo (Ed.), *Family Ethnicity* (pp. 90-108). Newbury Park, CA: Sage Publications.

Henderson, Dorothy J., Boyd, Carol, and Mieczkowski, Thomas (1994). "Gender, Relationships and Crack Cocaine: A Content Analysis." *Research in Nursing and Health* 117: 265-272.

Herskovits, Melville J. 1941. *The Myth of the Negro Past.* Boston: Beacon Press.

Hill Collins, Patricia. 1991. "Black Women and Motherhood." In Patricia Hill Collins (Ed.), *Black Feminist Thought* (pp. 115-138). New York: Routledge, Chapman and Hall, Inc.

Hill Collins, Patricia. 1994. "The Meaning of Motherhood in Black Culture." In Robert Staples (Ed.), *The Black Family,* Fifth edition (pp. 165-173). Belmont, CA: Wadsworth Publishing Company.

Hoffman, J. A., Klein, H., Eber, M., and Crosby, H. 2000. "Frequency and Intensity of Crack Use as Predictors of Women's Involvement in HIV-Related Sexual Risk Behaviors." *Drug and Alcohol Dependence* 58: 227-236.

hooks, bell. 1981. *Ain't I a Woman: Black Women and Feminism.* Boston: South End Press.

Inciardi, James A. 1989. "Trading Sex for Crack Among Juvenile Drug Users: A Research Note." *Contemporary Drug Problems* Winter: 689-700.

Inciardi, James. 1995. "Crack, Crack House Sex and HIV Risk." *Archives of Sexual Behavior* 24(3): 249-269.

Inciardi, James A., Lockwood, Dorothy, and Pottieger, Anne E. 1993. *Women and Crack Cocaine.* New York: Macmillan Publishing Company.

Inciardi, James A. and Surratt, Hilary. 2001. "Drug Use, Street Crime, and Sex-Trading among Cocaine Dependent Women: Implications for Public Health and Criminal Justice Policy." *Journal of Psychoactive Drugs* 33(4): 379-389.

Jackson, Jacquelyne. 1971. "But Where Are the Men?" In Robert Staples (Ed.), *The Black Family,* Second edition (pp. 110-117). Belmont, CA: Wadsworth Publishing Company.

Jacobs, Bruce A. 1999. *Dealing Crack: The Social World of Street Corner Selling.* Boston: Northeastern University Press.

Janesick, Valerie. 1998. "The Dance of Qualitative Research Design: Metaphor, Methodolatry and Meaning." In Norman K. Denzin and Yvonna S. Lincoln (Eds.), *Strategies of Qualitative Inquiry* (pp. 35-55). Thousand Oaks, CA: Sage Publications.

Jaret, Charles. 1986. "Black Migration and Socio-economic Inequality in Atlanta and the Urban South." *Humboldt Journal of Social Relations* 14(1-2): 62-105.

Johnson, Charles S. 1934. *The Shadow of the Plantation.* Chicago: University of Chicago Press.

Kanteowitz, Barbara. 1990. "The Crack Children." *Newsweek* 115(7): 62-63.

Kaplan, David W., Feinstein, Ronald A., Fisher, Martin M., Klein, Jonathan D., Olmedo, Luis F., Rome, Ellen S., Yancy, W. Samuel, Adams Hillard, Paula J., Pearson, Glen, Sacks, Diane, et al. 2001. American Academy of Pediatrics Committee on Adolescence and Committee on Early Childhood, Adoption, and Dependent Care. "Care of Adolescent Parents and Their Children." *Pediatrics* 107(2): 429-434.

Katz, William Lorenz. (Ed.). 1968. *Five Slave Narratives.* New York: Arno Press.

Kawachi, Ichiro. 1999. "Social Capital and Community Effects on Population and Individual Health." *Annals of the New York Academy of Sciences* 896(1): 120-130.

Kawachi, Ichiro and Kennedy, Bruce. 1997. "The Relationship of Income Inequality to Mortality: Does the Choice of Indicator Matter?" *Social Science and Medicine* 45(7): 1121-1127.

Kearney, Margaret H., Murphy, Sheigla, and Rosenbaum, Marsha. 1994a. "Learning by Losing: Sex and Fertility on Crack Cocaine." *Qualitative Health Research* 4(2): 142-162.

Kearney, Margaret H., Murphy, Shiegla, and Rosenbaum, Marsha. 1994b. "Mothering on Crack Cocaine: A Grounded Theory Analysis" *Social Science Medicine* 38(2): 351-361.

Kelley, Susan J. 1992. "Parenting Stress and Child Maltreatment in Drug Exposed Children." *Child Abuse and Neglect* 16: 317-328.

Kenen, Regina H. and Armstrong, Kay. 1992. "The Why and the Whether of Condom Use Among Female and Male Drug Users." *Journal of Community Health* 17(5): 303-317.

Kennedy, Bruce, Kawachi, Ichiro, Prothrow-Stith, Deborah, Lochner, Kimberly, and Gupta, Vanita. 1998. "Social Capital, Income Inequality and Firearm Violent Crime." *Social Science Medicine* 41(1): 7-17.

King, Patricia. 1991. "Helping Women Helping Children: Drug Policy and Future Generations." *The Milbank Quarterly* 69(4): 595-621.

Kreek, Mary Jeanne. 1998. "Neurobiological Correlates of the Addictions: Findings from Basic and Treatment Research." In *Drug Addiction Research and the Health of Women* (pp. 81-104). U. S. Department of Health and Human Services. National Institutes of Health National Institute on Drug Abuse.

Lewis, Diane K. 1977. "A Response of Inequality: Black Women, Racism and Sexism." In Malson, Madimbe-Boyi, O'Barr, and Wyer (Eds.), *Black Women in America*. Chicago: University of Chicago Press.

Lewis, Hylan. 1955. *Blackways of Kent.* New Haven, CT: College and University Press.

Lewis, Mary Ann, Giovannoni, Jeanne, and Leake, Barbara. 1997. "Ethic Variations in the Two Year Living Arrangements of Prenatally Drug Exposed and Comparison Children Placed at Birth." *Journal of Multicultural Social Work* 6(2): 17-40.

Lewis, Oscar. 1965. *La Vida.* New York: Random House.

Liebow, Elliot. 1967. *Tally's Corner.* New York: Little, Brown and Company.

Litt, Jacquelyn and McNeil, Maureen. 1997. "Biological Markers and Social Differentiation: Crack Babies and the Construction of the Dangerous Mother." *Health Care for Women International* 18: 31-41.

Mahan, Sue. 1996. *Crack Cocaine, Crime and Women: Legal Social and Treatment Issues.* London: Sage Publications.

Maher, Lisa. 1990. "Criminalizing Pregnancy: The Downside of a Kinder, Gentler Nation?" *Social Justice* 17(3): 111-135.

Maher, Lisa and Daly, Kathleen. 1996. "Women in the Street Level Drug Economy: Continuity or Change." *Criminology* 34(4): 465-491.

Mann, Susan. 1989. "Slavery, Sharecropping and Sexual Inequality." In Malson, Madimbe-Boyi, O'Barr, and Wyer (Eds.), *Black Women in America* (pp. 133-157). Chicago: University of Chicago Press.

Marques, Paul R. and McKnight, A. James. 1991. "Drug Abuse Risk Among Pregnant Adolescents Attending Public Health Clinics." *American Journal of Drug and Alcohol Abuse* 17(4): 399-413.

Marx, Rani, Aral, Sevgi, Rolfs, Robert, Sterk, Claire, and Kahn, James. 1990. "Crack, Sex and STD." *Sexually Transmitted Diseases* 18(2): 92-101.

Massey, Douglas and Denton, Nancy. 1999. "American Apartheid: The Perpetuation of the Underclass" In Charles Gallagher (Ed.), *Rethinking the Color Line* (pp. 316-336). Mountain View, CA: Mayfield Publishers.

McCoy, Clyde B., Metsch, Lisa R., Inciardi, James A., Anwyl, Robert S., Wingerd, Judith, and Bletzer, Keith. "Sex, Drugs and the Spread of HIV/AIDS in Belle Glad, Florida." *Medical Anthropology Quarterly* 10(1): 83-93.

Miller, Jody. 1995. "Gender and Power on the Streets: Street Prostitutes in the Era of Crack Cocaine." *Journal of Contemporary Ethnography* 23(4): 427-452.

Minkler, Meredith and Roe, Kathleen. 1993. *Grandmothers as Care Givers: Raising the Children of the Crack Cocaine Epidemic.* Newbury Park, CA: Sage Publications.

Minkler, Meredith, Roe, Kathleen, and Price, Marilyn. 1992. "The Physical and Emotional Health of Grandmothers Raising Grandchildren in the Crack Cocaine Epidemic." *The Gerontologist* 32(6): 752-761.

Moore, William, Jr. 1969. *The Vertical Ghetto.* New York: Random House.

Moynihan, Daniel P. 1965. *The Negro Family: The Case for National Action.* Washington, DC: U.S. Department of Labor.

Muller, Rachel Beaty and Boyle, Joyceen S. 1996. "You Don't Ask for Trouble: Women Who Do Sex and Drugs." *Family and Community Health* 19(3): 35-48.

Murphy, Sheigla B. and Rosenbaum, Marsha. 1997. "Two Women Who Used Cocaine Too Much: Class, Race, Gender, Crack and Coke." In Craig Reinarman and Harry Levine (Eds.), *Crack in America: Demon Drugs and Social Justice* (pp. 98-111). Berkeley: University of California Press.

Murray, Charles. 1984. *Losing Ground: American Social Policy 1950-1980.* New York: Basic Books, Inc.

Noel, Donald L. 1968. "A Theory of the Origin of Ethnic Stratification" In Norman Yetman (Ed.), *Majority and Minority* (pp. 113-124). Boston: Allyn & Bacon.

Omi, Michael and Winant, Howard. 1994. *Racial Formation in the United States: From the 1960s to the 1990s.* New York: Routledge Press.

Orfield, Gary and Ashkinaze, Carole. 1991. *The Closing Door: Conservative Policy and Black Opportunity.* Chicago: University of Chicago Press.

Palthrow, Lynn M. 1990. "When Becoming Pregnant Is a Crime." *Criminal Justice Ethics* 9: 41-47.

Palthrow, Lynn M. 1998. "Punishing Women for Their Behavior During Pregnancy: An Approach that Undermines the Health of Women and Children." In Cora Lee Wetherington and Adele Roman (Eds.), *Drug Addiction Research and the Health of Women* (pp. 467-501). National Institute on Drug Abuse Publication #98-4290. Bethesda, MD: National Institutes of Health.

Pursley-Crotteau, Suzanne and Stern, Phyllis Noerager. 1996. "Creating a New Life: Dimensions of Temperance in Perinatal Cocaine Crack Users." *Qualitative Health Research* 6(3): 350-367.

Putman, Robert. 2000. *Bowling Alone: The Collapse and Revival of American Community.* New York: Simon & Schuster.

Radecki, Stephen and Beckman, Linda. 1992. "Determinants of Child-Bearing Intentions of Low-Income Women: Attitudes Versus Life Circumstances." *Journal of Biosocial Science* 24: 157-166.

Rainwater, Lee. 1960. *And the Poor Get Children.* Chicago: Quadrangle Books.

Rainwater, Lee. 1970. *Behind Ghetto Walls.* Chicago: Aldine Publishing Company.

Ratner, Mitchell S. (Ed.). 1993. *Crack Pipe As Pimp.* New York: Lexington Books.

Robbins, James M. 1981. "Religious Asceticism and Abortion Among Low Income Black Women." *Sociological Analysis* 41(4): 365-374.

Rosenbaum, Marsha. 1981. *Women on Heroin*. New Brunswick, NJ: Rutgers University Press.

Rosenberg, Morris. 1965. *Society and the Adolescent Self Image*. Princeton, NJ: Princeton University Press.

Rosse, Richard, Fay-McCarthy, Maureen, Collins, Joseph, Risher-Flowers, Debra, Alim, Tanya, and Deutsch, Stephen. 1993. "Transient Compulsive Foraging Behavior Associated with Crack Cocaine Use." *American Journal of Psychiatry* 150(1): 155-156.

Rushton, J. Phillipe. 1996. "Race, Genetics, Human Reproductive Strategies." *Genetics, Social and General Psychological Monographs* 122: 21-53.

SAMHSA (Substance Abuse and Mental Health Services Administration). (2001). Results from the 2001 National Household Survey on Drug Abuse (NHSDA). Series H-17. Volume I. Summary of National Findings: 28. Rockville, MD: U.S. Department of Health and Human Services.

Sawicki, David and Moody, Mitch. 1997. "The Effects of Inter-Metropolitan Migration on the Labor Force Participation of Disadvantaged Black Men in Atlanta." *Economic Development Quarterly* 11(1): 45-66.

Schedler, George. 1992. "Forcing Pregnant Drug Addicts to Abort: Rights-Based and Utilitarian Justifications." *Social Theory and Practice* 18(3): 347.

Scheidweiler, K., Plessinger, M., Shojaie, J., Dwong, T., and Wood R. 1999. "Pharmaco-Kinetics of Methylegonidine, the Crack Pyrolysis Product." Paper presented at the College on Problems of Drug Dependence Annual Meeting in Acapulco, Mexico. June 1999. Rochester, NY: University of Rochester School of Medicine.

Schultz, David. 1978. "The Role of the Boyfriend in Lower-Class Negro Life." In Robert Staples (Ed.), *The Black Family* (pp. 72-76). Belmont, CA: Wadsworth Publishing Company.

Schwartzkopff, Frances. 1990. "Schools Brace for First Classes of 'Crack Kids.'" *Atlanta Journal-Constitution*. April 11: A1, A6.

Sharpe, Tanya T. 2001. "Sex for Crack Exchange, Poor Black Women and Pregnancy," *Qualitative Health Research* 11.5 (September): 612-630.

Siegel, Loren. 1997. "The Pregnancy Police Fight the War on Drugs." In Craig Reinarman and Harry Levine (Eds.), *Crack in America: Demon Drugs and Social Justice* (pp. 249-254) Berkeley: University of California Press.

Sowell, Thomas. 1994. *Race and Culture, A World View*. New York: Basic Books.

Stack, Carol. 1974. *All Our Kin: Strategies for Survival in a Black Community*. New York: Harper and Row.

Staples, Robert. 1970. "Educating the Black Male at Various Class Levels for Marital Roles." In Robert Staples (Ed.), *The Black Family* (pp. 167-171). Belmont, CA: Wadsworth Publishing Company.

Staples, Robert. 1971. "The Myth of the Impotent Black Male." In Robert Staples (Ed.), *The Black Family* (pp. 98-104). Belmont, CA: Wadsworth Publishing Company.

Staples, Robert (Ed). 1978. *The Black Family,* Second edition. Belmont, CA: Wadsworth Publishing Company.

Staples, Robert (Ed). 1986. *The Black Family,* Third edition. Belmont, CA: Wadsworth Publishing Company.

Staples, Robert. 1991a. "Changes in Black Family Structure: Conflict Between Family Ideology and Structural Conditions." In Robert Staples (Ed.), *The Black Family* (pp. 28-36). Belmont, CA: Wadsworth Publishing Company.

Staples, Robert. 1991b. "The Flip-Side of Black Families Headed by Women: The Economic Status of Black Men." In Robert Staples (Ed.), *The Black Family,* Fourth edition (pp. 117-123). Belmont, CA: Wadsworth Publishing Company.

Staples, Robert. 1991c. "Substance Abuse and the Black Family Crisis" In Staples, Robert (Ed.) *The Black Family* (pp. 257-267). Belmont, CA: Wadsworth Publishing Company.

Staples, Robert. 1994. *The Black Family,* Fifth edition. Belmont, CA: Wadsworth Publishing Company.

Stark, Rodney. 1994. *Sociology,* Fifth edition. Belmont, CA: Wadsworth, Inc.

Stephens, Richard. 1991. *The Street Addicts Role: A Theory of Heroin Addiction.* New York: State University of New York Press.

Sterk, Claire. 1988. "Cocaine and seropositivity." *The Lancet* (May 7): 1052-1053.

Sterk, Claire. 1990. *Living the Life: Prostitutes and Their Health.* Unpublished doctoral dissertation. City University of New York.

Sterk-Elifson, Claire and Elifson, Kirk W. 1993. "The Social Organization of Crack Cocaine Use: The Cycle in One Type of Base House." *Journal of Drug Issues* 23(3): 429-441.

Strauss, Anselm and Corbin, Juliet. 1990. *The Basics of Qualitative Research.* Newbury Park, CA: Sage Publications.

Strauss, Anselm and Glaser, B. 1967. *The Discovery of Grounded Theory.* Chicago: Aldine de Gruyter.

Subramanian, S. V., Lochner, Kimberly, and Kawachi, Ichiro. 2003. "Neighborhood Differences in Social Capital: A Compositional Artifact or a Contextual Construct?" *Health and Place* 9: 33-44.

Sudarkasa, Niara. 1993. "Female-Headed African-American Households: Some Neglected Dimensions." In Harriette Pipes McAdoo (Ed.), *Family Ethnicity* (pp. 81-89). Newbury Park, CA: Sage Publications.

Sudarkasa, Niara. 1996. *The Strengths of Our Mothers: African and African American Women and Families: Essays and Speeches.* Trenton, NJ: African World Press.

Thomas, Keith. 1986. "A New Form of Cocaine is Cracking the Drug Market in Atlanta." *Atlanta Journal-Constitution.* June 27: C1.

Toufexis, Anatasia. 1991. "Innocent Victims." *Time* 137(19): 56-60.

United States Department of Health and Human Services. 1997. Drug Abuse Warning Network Data (DAWN). Substance Abuse and Mental Health Services Administration (SAMHSA). Washington, DC: Office of Applied Studies.

United State Department of Health and Human Services. 2001. Drug and Alcohol Services Information System (DASIS). "Women in Treatment for Smoked Cocaine." Substance Abuse and Mental Health Services Administration (SAMHSA), July 13. Washington, DC: Office of Applied Studies.

United State Department of Health and Human Services. 2003. Drug Abuse Warning Network Data (DAWN). "Trends in Drug-Related Emergency Department Visits, 1994-2001 at a Glance." Substance Abuse and Mental Health Services Administration (SAMHSA).Washington, DC: Office of Applied Studies.

United State Department of Health and Human Services. 2005. Drug and Alcohol Services Information System (DASIS). "Smoked Cocaine vs. Non-Smoked Cocaine Admissions, 2002." Substance Abuse and Mental Health Services Administration (SAMHSA). February 25. Washington, DC: Office of Applied Studies.

Visser, Steve. 2002. "Sister Tells Horror of Boy's Abuse." Atlanta Journal-Constitution, December 12. Available online at: <http://www.gahsc.org/terrell/trial1 .html>.

Wacquant, Loic J. D. and Wilson, William Julius. 1991. "The Cost of Racial and Class Exclusion in the Inner City. Annals of the American Political and Social Science." In Norman R. Yetman (Ed.), *Majority and Minority: The Dynamics of Race and Ethnicity in American Life* (pp. 498-511). Boston: Allyn & Bacon.

Waldorf, Dan, Reinarman, Craig, and Murphy, Sheigla. 1991. *Cocaine Changes.* Philadelphia: Temple University Press.

Wallace, Barbara. 1991. *Crack Cocaine.* New York: Brunner/Mazel Publishers.

Ward, Martha C. 1986. *Poor Women, Powerful Men: America's Great Experiment in Family Planning.* Boulder: Westview Press.

Waterston, Alisse. 1993. *Street Addicts in the Political Economy.* Philadelphia: Temple University Press.

Williams, Terry. 1989. *The Cocaine Kids.* New York: Addison Wesley Publishing Company.

Wilson, William J. 1978. *The Declining Significance of Race.* Chicago: The University of Chicago Press.

Wilson, William J. 1987. *The Truly Disadvantaged.* Chicago: The University of Chicago Press.

Wilson, William J. 1996. *When Work Disappears.* Chicago: The University of Chicago Press.

Witkin, Gordon. 1991. "The Men Who Created Crack." *U. S. News and World Report* August 19: 44-53.

Wood, Ronald. 1999. "Michael Addition Reaction of the Crack Pyrolysis Product, Methylecgonidine in Pregnant Ewes." E-mail Correspondence, July 22, 1999. University of Rochester, Rochester, NY.

Wood, Ronald W., Graefe, J. F., Fang, C. P., Shojaie, Jalil, Chen, L. C., and Willetts, J. 1996a. "Generation of Stable Test Atmospheres of Cocaine Base and Its Pyrolysis Product, Methylecgonidine and Demonstration of Their Biological Activity." *Pharmacology Biochemistry and Behavior* 55(2): 237-248.

Wood, Ronald W., Shojaie, Jalil, Fang C. P., and Graefe, J. F. 1996b. "Methylecgonidine Coats the Crack Particle." *Pharmacology Biochemistry and Behavior* 53(1): 57-66.

Woods, James R. 1998. "Translating Basic Research on Drugs and Pregnancy into the Clinical Setting." In Cora Lee Wetherington and Adele Roman (Eds.), *Drug Addiction Research and the Health of Women* (pp. 187-195). National Institute on Drug Abuse Publication #98-4290. Bethesda, MD: National Institutes of Health.

Young, Amy, Boyd, Carol, and Hubbell, Amy. 2000. "Prostitution, Drug Use, and Coping with Psychological Distress." *Journal of Drug Issues* 30(4): 789-800.

Index

Page numbers followed by the letter "t" indicate tables; those followed by the letter "f" indicate figures.